Heartbreaker

Heartbreaker

Christiaan Barnard and the first heart transplant

James-Brent Styan

Jonathan Ball Publishers
JOHANNESBURG & CAPE TOWN

Originally published in South Africa in 2017 by
JONATHAN BALL PUBLISHERS
A division of Media24 (Pty) Ltd
PO Box 33977
Jeppestown
2043

ISBN 978- 1-86842-842-7
ebook ISBN 978- 1-86842-843-4

Twitter: www.twitter.com/JonathanBallPub
Facebook: www.facebook.com/JonathanBallPublishers
Blog: http://jonathanball.bookslive.co.za/
Cover by Michiel Botha
Cover photograph: David Goldblatt / South Photographs /
Africa Media Online
Design and typesetting by Triple M Design
Set in 11/15pt Sabon MT Pro

Printed by *paarlmedia*, a division of Novus Holdings

This is for my mother, Jurina.
She was a Karoo girl.

I remember how we followed Chris Barnard's story
in the Huisgenoot. *You would have enjoyed the story again.*
We miss you terribly.

Contents

Prologue

Cape Town, Saturday evening, 2 December 1967

IT WAS LATE EVENING WHEN THE PHONES STARTED RINGING ALL ACROSS the Cape Peninsula. Amelia 'Pittie' Rautenbach, Sannie Rossouw and Tollie Lambrechts were at a costume party in the Cape Town suburb of Mowbray. The three scrub sisters were dressed in 1920s-era bathing suits – a sensible choice for a warm, December evening in Cape Town.

'We were all very jolly and had already had a few drinks. No-one could've expected us to sit there the whole night without having a drink,' says Rossouw.

Lambrechts, who was hosting the party, says they'd been drinking punch but hadn't even got to the fruity bits yet when the phone rang and they got the message. The three women dropped everything and ran.

'We were just told we must come, there's a donor,' says Lambrechts.[1]

They drove to Groote Schuur in two cars. Rossouw had no opportunity to change from her bathing suit, so she went into the operating theatre wearing her costume under her theatre scrubs.

'Everyone was so busy with their own tasks, no-one even noticed it.'[2]

That night a team of 30 people were called in for an operation that would bring the world to a standstill – the world's first human-to-human heart transplant.

It would be an operation that would represent a quantum leap in medical science and one which would open up a Pandora's box of controversies, including the question – when is a person actually dead?

To have any chance of success, the team doing the operation had to be world-class. The transplant team had been on 24-hour standby for three weeks, while the heart unit waited for a donor heart. It had been a long time coming, but this Saturday evening, the long wait was over for the three theatre sisters and their 25 colleagues. The final step to the summit of the medical world's Everest could be taken.

The world would awaken to the news that a medical team from Groote Schuur Hospital in Cape Town had performed the first successful human-to-human heart transplant. For the world, it was an unexpected medical accomplishment, achieved by unsung and unknown outsiders and against the run of play. It was to be an accomplishment achieved by people relying on a tiny percentage of the budget compared to similar programmes in countries like America where heart transplantation was being compared with the race to land a man on the moon.

For the leader of the Groote Schuur team, the operation was a tremendous personal risk. If the operation was a disaster, his medical career might be over forever: he might even face murder charges. It would take enormous courage and self-confidence to cut out one patient's sick – but still beating – heart and replace it with a donor heart.

Later in his life, the leader of the surgical team that had changed history, wrote about the famous general Hannibal Barca, who crossed the Alps using elephants to transport supplies.

'History remembers Hannibal as a genius. But only because he won. Had the result turned out differently, he would have been remembered as a damn fool.'

That writer and the surgeon behind the scalpel was Christiaan Barnard.

PART ONE

In the beginning, 1922–1967

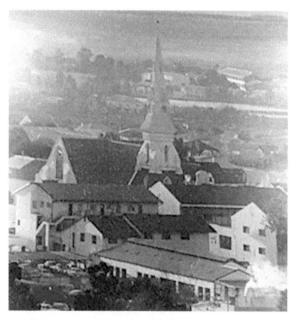

The Karoo town of Beaufort West with the church steeple standing tall in the centre of town.

PHOTOGRAPH COURTESY OF THE 318 AMANDA BOTHA COLLECTION,

DOCUMENT CENTRE, STELLENBOSCH UNIVERSITY

CHAPTER I

Sons of the Karoo

Adam

EVEN THOUGH ADAM HENDRIKUS BARNARD HAD A DRIVER'S LICENCE, he refused to drive. This was a final, conscious decision taken the day he missed his turn off to 77 Donkin Street and ended up careering through the front door of the missionary church in Beaufort West. By this time, grey-haired Adam had had a long and nail-biting history behind the wheel of his black Model T Ford, but landing his car between the pine benches in the church was the final straw that broke the camel's back.[1] He decided, then and there, to lay off driving and never touch a steering wheel again. The slender, thin-moustached Adam was about 70 years old, with a face full of wrinkles and furrows that replicated the landscape of his beloved Karoo. But he had started life as far removed from the arid Karoo of Beaufort West as one can get in South Africa.

Adam grew up in the majestic Knysna forests in the 1800s, under gigantic yellowwood trees, with wild elephants and bright green and red Knysna bosloeries for company. He was one of eight children of a dirt-poor woodcutter family, descendants of a German soldier who had stepped ashore in Cape Town in 1708. The soldier married a Dutch immigrant's daughter and the couple had two sons and a daughter. Every Barnard in South Africa today is a descendant of the second son. The first son had no offspring.[2]

Adam's story is remarkably similar to that of the main character in

Dalene Matthee's novel, *Circles in a Forest*, published in 1984. The fictional story of Saul Barnard's life in the Knysna forest could just as well have been Adam Barnard's story. The fictional Saul and the living Adam shared three distinct characteristics while growing up: both led deeply religious lifestyles, and both lacked education and lived in acute poverty.

Families living in the Knysna forest struggled on a daily basis to stay alive, never mind make ends meet.[3] The forest people were also known for their seclusion from the outside world. Most of them simply never left – they were born and raised in the forest, and they died there.

But the young Adam was an exception. He had aspirations to improve himself and see the outside world, so he left the family business and ventured forth into the great unknown as an uneducated outsider.

His youngest son, Marius, would later say that this image of his father leaving the Knysna forest, and the enormous implications of this decision, became a defining memory in Marius's life.[4]

Adam's new life started in the Salvation Army, where he served selflessly and with distinction for some time, including a period in the Anglo-Boer War. Along the way he picked up a debilitating illness and, following a range of physical check-ups, it was decided he could no longer continue in the Salvation Army. At this stage Adam recognised the limitations placed on him by his lack of education, so when he was 23 years old he went to study at the NG Kerk missionary school in Wellington. When he was asked where he would like to start, he simply replied, 'At the beginning.'

While Adam was still a student, he went on a practical training course in the district of Joubertina. There he met Maria de Swardt, a tall and attractive brunette from a family of relatively well-off farmers, ironically from the George area. Maria had been doing practical nursing training in the same district as Adam. Her background was very different from that of the forest people and the only thing the two had in common was religion. Over weekends she played the organ in the local church in town and this is where they met.

The De Swardt family viewed the relationship in a rather poor light, believing that Adam was below Maria's class – a poor forest dweller.[5] The couple were unfazed, however, and following a short courtship – and to the horror of Maria's family – the two got married.

Two years later Adam completed his studies. After four years of study, graduates had a choice to work either as teachers or as missionaries.[6] For Adam, the choice was simple: he was always going to become a missionary. His background, together with his experiences in the Salvation Army, particularly the belief in serving others regardless of race or status, would serve him well into the future. 'Love Thy Neighbour' would become not only a theological concept but a way of life. His life was characterised by his unceasing support and love for the poor, the downtrodden and the desperate, across all racial lines, even during the darkest days of apartheid. This would often come at huge personal cost.

After a few years of moving around, including a stint in Graaff-Reinet, the Barnards settled in Beaufort West in 1911 where Adam became the missionary in charge of the local mission church – the very same church into which he would later crash his Model T Ford.

Beaufort West

The Barnards settled into the stately old missionary parsonage on the same plot of land as the missionary church. The address was originally 77 Donkin Street but in later years it was changed to number 91. There was a small rose garden in front of the house, while the backyard was a large empty piece of land where Adam and Maria's four sons spent their youth.

As Johannes Barnard, the eldest of the four Barnard sons, recalled in later years to *Die Burger* newspaper, 'There were fruit trees and vineyards as well as neat garden beds where my parents grew vegetables. There was a large, old oak tree and a lemon tree.'

During those early years, barely 10 years after the Anglo-Boer War, the South African countryside was still recovering from the devastating turmoil that had created large divisions within South Africa and destroyed large segments of the population. The countryside was a place for tough and hardened people, used to hard work and struggling to make ends meet.[7]

Afrikaner Nationalism was gaining a foothold across the country – a nationalism founded on self-identity and a hatred of all things English. Perhaps as a result of there being few English people in the countryside, there was a growing focus on nationalism and discrimination in terms of race. Beaufort West was also a deeply divided town in those days.

The Gamka River – in reality a dry river bed rather than an actual river – which cuts through the town, became a racial border that divided the town into two. On the one side of the Gamka was the white *bodorp* ('upper town') with the business centre, the magistrates' court and the post office. This is where the large houses of the wealthier white people were situated. On the other side of the river, in an area with no electricity and very few other facilities, were the small shacks and informal dwellings of the coloured community. The 7 000 or so people who lived in this part of town were Adam's congregation for the next 37 years of his life.

The racial tensions were worsened by the First World War. In South Africa at the time, many Afrikaners were extremely unhappy with the government because of its decision to enter the war on the side of the English. This discontent led to a failed rebellion by some Afrikaners.

In Beaufort West, the tension was also palpable. What made matters worse for the Barnards was the fact that they were one of very few white families in the district that were not on the side of Germany. The largely German-allied whites in the town often made their feelings towards the Barnard family very clear.

At this time, Johannes was four years old. He was one of twins but his sister was stillborn. 'I remember one evening when a large crowd marched up and down the main road singing and dancing. My father told me they were happy because the Germans were busy winning the war,' says Johannes.

After Johannes, Adam and Maria had another four children, all boys: Dodsley, Abraham, Christiaan and Marius. Johannes is quoted as saying that as a youngster during the war he was terrified of what would happen to him and his parents if the Germans were to win.[8]

Tragedy hit the family when Abraham died of a heart condition before his third birthday, despite all his parents' efforts to save him, including taking him to Cape Town for treatment at huge expense. On the night of Abraham's death, Adam sat next to him and tried to soothe him by feeding him bits of a Marie biscuit and cleaning his nails with a matchstick. Abraham died in the Cape Town suburb of Muizenberg and was buried there. The matchstick and tooth-marked biscuit were all that Adam had left to remember his son; that and a photograph of the boy that would hang in the lounge.[9]

Christiaan and Marius would later explain that their brother had probably died as result of a hole in the heart – a condition that is easily fixed today but which was irreparable at the time.

In addition to the stress relating to the townspeople, Maria struggled to get over the death of her two young children. Their deaths remained with her for the rest of her life and cast a sad shadow over the family. Maria also became increasingly conservative in her religion and after Abraham's death she wore mainly black. She also changed emotionally and started having angry outbursts, many of which were aimed at Johannes. This often meant an irrational hiding, often with a heavy hairbrush. Johannes recalled that she got worse and worse and often punished him for the smallest thing.

Then Christiaan was born and he would become the apple of his mother's eye.

Christiaan Barnard

The Barnard family had no money to get a doctor for the birth, so Christiaan Neethling Barnard was helped into the world on 8 November 1922 by a midwife whose surname was Neethling.

At the time of Christiaan's birth – the family called him Chrisjan – Beaufort West was still little more than a sheep-farming community and a stopover between Johannesburg and Cape Town. However, the townspeople were proud of their large church – the largest building in Beaufort West – with its beautiful tower topped by an imposing cast-iron weathervane. This impressive church tower with its large bell could be seen from kilometres around and was a beacon to travellers approaching the town. The *Boerekerk* – also known as the *Moederkerk* – with its beautiful wooden carvings and decorated ceiling high above the rafters was a hospitable meeting place for its congregants. This church, led by Dominee Rabie, served the 3 400 white families from the district.

In comparison, Adam's missionary church was much more basic. It had no tower or bell, just a small organ and plain pine benches.

The two churches were in the main road of the town, not much more than 50 metres apart,[10] but the separation might as well have been 100 kilometres. The coloured community attending Adam's church was not allowed to attend the *Boerekerk*, and whites – except for the Barnards – did not attend Adam's church.

The two shepherds' circumstances were different in almost every way, because even though the townsfolk lived in the same place, served the same God and even sang the same hymns, the colour of their skin was different. While Adam tended to his flock in their ramshackle wood-and-iron shacks on the one side of the semi-desert town, Dominee Rabie often dined at the tables of congregants living in the biggest houses and best farms in the district.

The Barnard sons did not have things easy. According to Johannes, 'There was never enough food. Although the four of us would never starve, we were often hungry. Mom would keep the pantry locked between meals. She was quite frugal and would measure off each day's food quota carefully – so much sugar, so much rice and so forth. When the day's food was finished, there was nothing more till the next morning. Often the garden would help us out. In season, we boys would find corn, beans and tomatoes, which we would eat raw. In the winter when everything was gone, there was a lemon tree that helped. We would eat the sour fruit, peel and all.'[11]

Adam wasn't a minister or a parson. Instead his official title was the much less important one of reverend because he had been sent by the

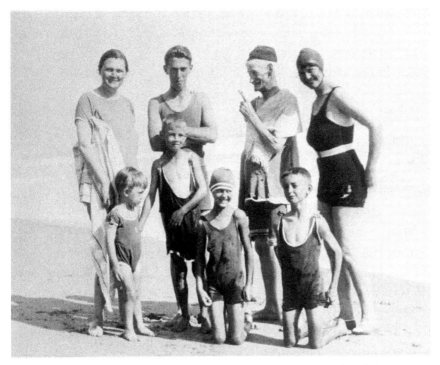

Barnard family portrait taken in 1930. Standing at the back, from left to right, are Maria Barnard, Johannes Barnard, Adam Barnard and a family friend. In the front from left to right are Marius Barnard, Christiaan Barnard and two friends. Dodsley Barnard is not pictured.

PHOTOGRAPH COURTESY OF THE HEART OF CAPE TOWN MUSEUM.

church as a missionary. For his missionary work, Reverend Barnard was paid R40 per month, while Dominee Rabie was paid R120 per month.

To earn a little extra, Adam would get up early every Sunday morning and walk over three kilometres to the jail outside town, where he would preach the gospel of love to the souls incarcerated behind bars. For this additional effort, Adam received a further R3 per month. Often Adam sacrificed his own annual leave to work in the white *Boerekerk* for extra income when Dominee Rabie went on holiday.

His work with the prisoners often led to a knock at the back door of the family home when prisoners were released and were in need of help.

Most often the help that was needed was money to enable them to travel to their homes, often in far-off areas. Others wanted cash to have a drink – and some were quite honest about it! Adam would chase them away empty-handed with a fiery sermon about the evils of alcohol.

Matriarch

Christiaan and his brothers rarely got anything new and clothes were never a priority. The boys would rely on hand-me-downs, often passing a piece of clothing down from the eldest to the youngest.[12]

Maria, who was an excellent seamstress, also made sure her sons had clothes. Her fabric of choice was the rough khaki of the time, from which she would make her sons pairs of shorts and shirts.[13] The Barnard boys felt that it was important to have pockets in their shorts but to save material Maria would only allow them only one per pair. The family joke was that the boys could choose on which side their pocket should be – as long as it was the right-hand side![14]

Maria often helped out as organist in the *Boerekerk* for extra income but the problem was that she was hard of hearing. Things got so bad in later years that she couldn't hear when the dominee announced a hymn. To overcome this challenge, Maria roped in her younger son – first Christiaan and later Marius. When the time came for Maria to play, her son would give her a light bump and then the sounds of *Rock of Ages* or *Onward Christian Soldiers* would break out.

The racial discrimination in the conservative rural town was at a high when Christiaan and Marius were youngsters. There was even an evening curfew for all people classified as 'non-whites'. When the clock – the one at the top of the *Boerekerk* steeple – rang at 9.00pm, they all had to be out of the *bodorp*.[15]

The townspeople looked down on the four Barnard sons because of the work their father was doing among the coloured community.[16] 'Father's calling was often rubbed in our faces. We quickly became known as the sons of the *hotnot predikant*. It was a term not only deriving from the fact that Father was a missionary, but also because we were poor and always poorly dressed. We never had money to spend like the children of the rich wool farmers and some other townspeople.'[17]

The boys were often discriminated against because their father shook the hands of coloured people. As a youngster, Christiaan could never understand the laws of his country: 'These rules said people were not the same, but because of the colour of their skin, they were different.'[18]

Although Adam had his hands full with the poor community he was serving, he always had time to love his children. At the same time, his work meant that Maria had to oversee all other aspects of the boys' upbringing, including their education.

Maria has been described as a hard and tough woman; one filled with ruthless ambition for her boys, whom she would beat if they didn't finish first in class. As a youngster, Chris would often have to scrub the floors of the family home. No matter how long and hard he did it, it was never good enough for his mother. Maria always pushed Christiaan hard to be first; second was never an option.[19]

'My Chris could always manage to do what other children found too difficult,' she said once.[20]

Christiaan was always her favourite and got away with more than his brothers did. For them, Maria had less mercy. Once Marius didn't come first in class and his mother beat him with a hairbrush; it was a hiding he never forgot.

Maria was a good wife and loved her family, but she was a cold and emotionless woman. There can be no doubt about Adam and Maria's commitment to each other. Although the boys never doubted this bond, they also never experienced their parents showing any affection, like a kiss or a hug.

Marius believed that his mother's lack of warmth was due to her orthodox upbringing and her bad hearing, which increasingly led to her being cut off from the outside world. In later years, one of her daughters-in-law said that although she had taught her sons well and had instilled great ambition in them, she had never taught them to understand the concept of love.[21]

Growing up in a parsonage as the sons of devout Calvinist parents, most things were considered to be sinful: drinking, smoking and dancing were evil incarnate and to be avoided at any cost.

Beaufort West organised dances in the city hall on Friday evenings (for whites only, of course) when Christiaan was in high school and just beginning to be interested in women. He was forbidden to go.

'My mother believed that dancing was the quickest way to hell,' Christiaan recalled later.[22]

As a 16-year-old, Christiaan knew that no girl would ever look twice at a guy who didn't dance, never mind one who wasn't even allowed to go to a dance, so he improvised and tricked his parents.[23]

'On Fridays, my curfew was 10.00pm, so I played the Cinderella thing. I would leave the house at 7.00pm, not dressed up at all, and go to a friend's house where I would dress up smartly and comb my hair. At the dance, I would meet my best girl and dance till the clock struck 10.00pm. Then it was a mad rush running back home. It was always very bad to leave while the music was still playing.'

Still, the boys grew up with very little knowledge of women and Marius learnt about menstruation only when he was at university.[24] Maria's influence on Christiaan during his formative years may have been the cause of his perceived emotional shallowness towards women in his later years.

Sons of the Karoo

For the young Barnard brothers, the Karoo was a magical place filled with wonderful things. Adam would often take his sons into the dry veld to camp under the bright stars. The old forester Adam taught his sons about nature and how to hunt using an ancient 18-gauge shotgun. They would hunt springhares in the moonlight and look for creatures under the rocks. In the winter Adam would show his dexterity with an axe and chop up the wood needed to feed the family's hungry Esse stove.

Christiaan always remembered his father on the pulpit. 'He had a white moustache and green-brown eyes. He looked like an eagle staring from his nest into a far-off valley.'[25]

Their father also taught Christiaan and Marius to hate racial discrimination. For years Adam waged a one-man war against the racial discrimination in the town. Despite racial anger and strong opposition, his hard-headedness and work led to the establishment of schools for the coloured community of Beaufort West. The primary school opened in 1931 in Bird Street in the centre of town.[26]

Adam became the superintendent of both the primary and high schools serving the coloured community in the town and accordingly played a substantial role in appointing teachers in both schools. The teachers were all coloured and were often better qualified and more experienced than their colleagues in the white schools in the town. This upset Adam's detractors even further, to such an extent that the townsfolk decided that the coloured primary school and the missionary church – which were in the centre of the town – had to be moved to the coloured area on the outskirts of town.

Again, Adam took up the fight to stop this plan. Although the local authorities tried everything to make the move happen, Adam managed to block them each time. On one occasion the town's leaders declared a special town by-law ordering the move, which would have made it compulsory. However, when Adam heard this, he took the first train to Cape Town, at his own cost, to petition the high court for an interdict against the ordinance. Once again he succeeded and the church and school were able to remain.

Sadly, Adam's struggle was eventually lost: the town's leaders simply waited patiently until he retired.

'At the age of 74, long after most people had already done so, Father retired. At that stage, he had been a missionary in Beaufort West for 37 years,' recalls Johannes.[27]

With his retirement, the road was clear and there was little resistance to the town's plans. In 1953 Excelsior Primary School was moved to the coloured area, where it was attended by coloured and black children. The school was moved again in 1962 due to the Group Areas Act, this time to Rustdene, where it remains today, renamed as the AH Barnard Primary School.

Adam's missionary church in the centre of town, was closed in 1964 and the church and parsonage were sold to the municipality for R40 000. Between 1967 and 1975 the church was used as a sporting hall for badminton.[28] The artefacts – few that there were – of the church were stripped and removed during the 1970s. Much later, following Christiaan's anger at the turn of events, things changed again and, in 1980, the church and parsonage were declared a national monument.[29]

The life of a son of the Karoo had other pros and cons. One of the pros was the local bioscope or cinema where the boys were able to watch the Saturday afternoon shows for four pence. The cinema brought the wonders of the world to Beaufort West and the boys watched the stories of Tarzan, played by Johnny Weissmuller, and Roy Rogers, to say nothing of the various female movie stars. It was a world far removed from the arid Karoo town where, at times, life weighed heavily on the innocent sons of the *hotnot predikant*.

Few would ever have guessed that barely 20 years later, Christiaan would become involved in passionate and scandalous affairs with movie stars whom he once would have been able to adore only from afar in the Star Cinema in Beaufort West.

Mortality

Eventually it was the death of Abraham – a brother he never knew – that had a profound impact on Christiaan, one that would drive him to achieving the impossible.

'Each of us can recall the moment when mortality became a reality for us for the first time. A moment when we suddenly realised that life ends. I recall it as a featherlike coolness that caressed my face softly when I was told that my baby brother had died and I felt that I had lost something. I guess that from that moment, death was a bold, concrete reality that would form a part of my life forever. Perhaps my childhood was over from that moment when I realised that life has an end,' Christiaan wrote in later years.[30]

Life would take Christiaan Barnard far away from the dusty streets of Beaufort West. His first destination was Cape Town, 461 kilometres to the south west along the N1 highway.

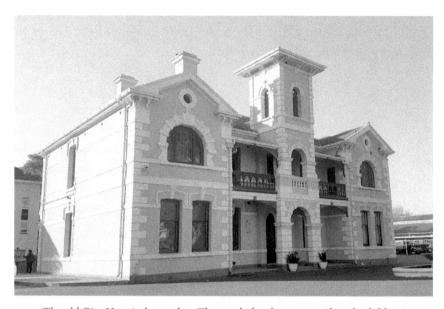

*The old City Hospital complex. The wards for the patients (largely children)
from poor communities with infectious diseases such as tuberculosis,
diphtheria, measles, scarlet fever and meningitis are behind this building.*

CHAPTER 2

Genius

IN 1940 CHRISTIAAN BARNARD ARRIVED IN CAPE TOWN TO STUDY MEDICINE at the University of Cape Town (UCT).[1] At the time, cardiology and heart surgery were still largely unknown and, in essence, non-existent. There was not much that could be done for patients with serious heart diseases.

Doctors across the world were loath to touch the human heart. One of the biggest stumbling blocks was the emotions associated with the organ. For millennia, the heart had been thought of as the foundation of the body, a mysterious organ that held within it the key to human emotion and intelligence – the home of the human soul. Despite the many medical advances over the centuries, by the Second World War it was almost unheard of to operate on a human heart.

In fact, before the war, there was only one reported case of an operation performed on a human heart. This report related to an incident in Frankfurt, Germany, in 1896 when a drunk man was assaulted and stabbed in the heart. He was taken to hospital with a wound the staff realised they couldn't treat. The patient, who was increasingly struggling to breathe, was in luck because the chief surgeon at the Frankfurt City Hospital was Ludwig Rehn.[2]

Rehn realised that the patient's heart membrane or pericardium was filling with blood from the wound in the heart and filling the space between the heart and the tough sinewy pericardium membrane that encases the heart. Blood was filling the space needed by the heart to pump blood around the body, thus limiting blood flow and making breathing increasingly difficult. Rehn took a great risk and cut open the pericardium membrane – a procedure that was unheard of in those days. The dammed-up blood spurted out in a thick stream as the pressure was relieved. Rehn observed the heart beating in the patient's chest and saw that tiny drops of blood were leaking out with each beat. He placed a finger on the hole to stop the bleeding, but it constantly slid off the slippery, fast-beating organ. He persisted, however, and stitched up the hole with three stitches. Two hours later, the patient awoke and was comfortable. This would become the first reported successful operation done on a human heart – three stitches.

However, Rehn was wary of taking his breakthrough much further than writing up the procedure and publishing it. His fear – shared by most doctors at the time – was that he might be the cause of the death of a patient and that the accompanying judgement by the professional fraternity might end his career.[3] His finger-in-the-dyke procedure was, however, a major stepping stone in changing perceptions around heart surgery.

The student communist

Christiaan Barnard's studies were made possible thanks to the financial support of the Helpmekaar Fonds, a fund established to assist Afrikaner children with financial difficulties with their academic studies.[4] Later this fund also helped to pay for Marius's studies. However, the fund covered only a portion of the total cost. The tuition fees were £60 per year and Christiaan received only £20 per annum from the fund; the balance was paid by Adam and Maria at great personal sacrifice.[5] He later received an additional £20 per annum from other bursaries at UCT.

Needless to say, there was no money for any extras. This meant that Christiaan had to stay with his eldest brother, Johannes, and his wife in a tiny flat in Rustenburg Road in Rosebank, Cape Town. He moved into a room under the eaves.[6]

In those days, first-year medical students had four subjects: chemistry, physiology, biology and zoology. For a country boy like Christiaan, physiology and chemistry were very tough and he had to spend long hours mastering these subjects. His financial situation meant that he could not afford to fail a subject, so he spent most of his student years studying.

Christiaan did manage to make a few friends, however, one of whom was Harry Khan, a fellow medical student, who had a great impact on his life. Harry was a self-confessed member of the Communist Party[7] and the two whiled away many hours debating religion and politics.

'We agreed that the average Joe in South Africa deserved a better life. That included non-whites. The treatment of non-white doctors was a disgrace, but we felt that the way non-whites were treated all over the country had to change,' Christiaan wrote later.

He continued: 'The trouble lay in the economic system. The profit motive led to people being seen as instruments rather than people. Wars were being declared to enrich a handful of people, while the young people of many nations died in the process. There was too much money in the hands of too few people.'

It may have been Christiaan's personal experiences of the white middle class in Beaufort West, who had wanted to shut down his father's church, that fired up his emotions.

'You agree with Karl Marx, then,' Harry said to Christiaan one day.

'I do?'

'Yes, you agree on issues like the wicked concentration of wealth in the hands of a few, the lack of political rights for the oppressed working class, war as a weapon of capitalism, the use of money to pervert the nature of labour, the plundering of people's dignity and identity through labour, the exploitation of the underprivileged non-whites and the selling out by the middle class to the owners of the industrial revolution,' Harry explained.

'Does that make me a communist?'

'Yes.'

'I don't know, I've never read Marx and never even known a real communist,' Christiaan said.

Harry started taking him along to meetings of the Communist Party, which was active at UCT, and Christiaan seriously considered joining the party.

'The manifesto of Marx tackled real problems and provided actual proposals for action and restructuring. It was very attractive,' Christiaan recalled in his later writings.

At about this time, Johannes and his wife bought a house in Pinelands and Christiaan moved in with them.[8] There was no bus or train service from Pinelands to UCT, which meant that the young student had to walk approximately 13 kilometres to and from classes. It was often an unpleasant experience, especially when the weather was bad. One relationship with a sweetheart named Jackie took a nosedive when she and another male student drove past a sopping wet Christiaan who was trudging along in the rain.

Christiaan's interest in communism ended when he had a falling-out with Harry regarding religion.

Harry told Chris: 'God is dead. He doesn't exist. Karl Marx was correct, religion is the opiate of the masses.'

Christiaan remembers the story as follows:

'Marx actually meant that religion was being used as a drug, but at that stage all I could think of was my father's love for God and how integral it was to his love for people. It was suddenly clear that Harry and I would never really agree.'

He said to Harry, 'So you're saying my dad is a drug peddler?'

'Sorry Chris, I didn't mean it like that,' Harry replied.

'That's okay.'

But it wasn't okay and the two students never discussed Marx again, or Christiaan joining the Communist Party.[9]

'My dad's life was not for nothing. He did not love a dead image. God was alive for him and for me.'

Christiaan had a distressing experience when he was in his fourth year of medical studies, the year in which the students started working with actual patients in the hospital. His first patient was an old woman with severe rheumatoid arthritis.

'She was in her 60s, terribly malformed and unable to get out of bed.

She could no longer use her hands or feet,' he recalled.[10]

The woman's condition upset him and haunted him for a long time afterwards. He had no idea of the impact the sickness would have on his life in later years.[11]

Louwtjie

One afternoon the young Christiaan visited a sick friend in Hall C2 at Groote Schuur. In the adjacent bed was a young nursing student named Louwtjie,[12] who asked Christiaan to post a letter to her family. He couldn't get over her exquisite hands.

Aletta Gertrude Louw had grown up in Mariental in South West Africa (now Namibia), probably the farthest one could get from city life – even more off the beaten track than Beaufort West. The attractive brunette was one of a close-knit family of five sisters and one brother named Tienie.[13] Her parents were among the first to farm valuable Karakul sheep in Namibia, but later, following the death of Tienie, they changed to cattle farming in the Okahandja district in central Namibia.

Tienie died tragically at the age of 25 following a rugby match in which he was kicked in the stomach. He died the following day of peritonitis and his death hit the family hard.[14]

Louwtjie had arrived at Groote Schuur when she was 18 years old to be trained in nursing. She was in her third year when she met Christiaan in Hall C2.

'Chris was a normal man but caring. He was ambitious, filled with a lust for life and determined to be a success. We were two simple youngsters from the countryside who met one another by accident and fell in love. The fact that Chris was an irresistible attraction for women is not in doubt and I was no exception,' Louwtjie wrote in her memoir.[15]

The couple became an item and dated for a few years.

It took Christiaan the normal six years to qualify as a medical doctor; six years of hardship and 13-kilometre walks carrying books and lunch tins, followed by nights spent alone in the medical laboratories at UCT.[16]

At the age of 24 years, Christiaan graduated with Louwtjie and his parents by his side.

It was at this time, in the late 1940s, shortly after the Second World War, that general thoracic surgery was being established as a specialty in South Africa. The programme was started in two centres, Cape Town and Durban. This medical field included lung and throat surgery and very limited work on the heart. The chief focus was on treating tuberculosis and penetrating trauma to the chest.[17]

House doctor in Ceres

Tim O'Maloney was the doctor in the little town of Ceres, about two hours' drive from Cape Town. He decided to take a long sabbatical and needed someone to take care of his practice while he was gone. He approached one of Christiaan's fellow students, Erhard 'Pikkie' Joubert, who agreed to take care of the practice in the old doctor's absence.[18]

Joubert quickly realised that there was too much work in Ceres for one doctor, so he invited Christiaan to join him. Christiaan found the offer attractive because he was planning marry Louwtjie. The position meant more money and job security, even though it wasn't exactly what he had been planning – his interest still lay in research work.[19] He eventually went to the Boland town to join Pikkie, without Louwtjie.

The two young doctors had a wonderful time in Ceres. They worked hard and became popular with the townsfolk. The practice grew and it became evident that by the time O'Maloney returned there would be enough room for all three doctors.

Two years later, on 6 November 1948 – a clear sunny day – Christiaan married Louwtjie in the Groote Kerk in Cape Town. Marius was the best man.[20]

'The two of them hired formal wear for the wedding. Marius's trousers were too long and he had to keep pulling up his pants,' Louwtjie recalls. [21]

After the photos were taken, the reception was held at a local eatery, the Koffiehuis, next to the church. Eric Crichton, a UCT professor in gynaecology and obstetrics, who had been one of Christiaan's early mentors, proposed the toast to the bridal couple. He also had some wisdom for Louwtjie.

'Prof Crichton whispered to me that I had to accept Christiaan was a committed and hardworking doctor. He said I would have to accept that his patients and his work would always come first and I would come second,' Louwtjie recalls.[22]

The couple spent two weeks on honeymoon in Wilderness near George after which they settled in Ceres.[23] To Christiaan's surprise he enjoyed the work and the position in the countryside. He learnt quickly how lonely it could be having to make life and death decisions.

Christiaan and Louwtjie's first child, Deirdre, was born on 28 April 1950. Later Louwtjie would report that the two years they lived in Ceres were the happiest of their married life.

But it couldn't last. And it didn't. Christiaan and Dr O'Maloney didn't get along. Professional jealousy reared its head as patients increasingly went to Christiaan for treatment rather than to the older doctor. The jealousy and anger grew to the point where the old doctor asked Christiaan to leave.

Christiaan was very angry, and even more so when his friend Pikkie seemed to choose O'Maloney's side over his. This was a severe blow after all the hard work the two of them had put into building the practice.

Initially Chris opened his own practice in the town but the townsfolk were loyal to Dr O'Maloney and, increasingly, the Barnards struggled financially. It was the NG Kerk dominee in the town who was Christiaan's one true pillar of support during this trying time. He advised Christiaan to desist from opposing his former colleagues.

His advice was well received and the Barnard family decided to move back to Cape Town, tail tucked firmly between their legs, and under uncertain circumstances.[24] They moved into a flat in the Strand owned by Louwtjie's parents. This was where André, the second child, was born on 30 March 1951.[25] Christiaan was unemployed at the time and this was a particularly stressful period for the family with two small children.

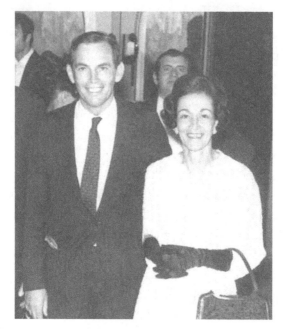

*The doctor who married the nurse. Chris and Louwtjie in a photograph
taken in the latter years of their relationship.*

Tuberculous meningitis

Salvation came when Christiaan saw a post advertised in the *South
African Medical Journal*. It was at the City Hospital for Infectious
Diseases, an institution in Portswood Road in Green Point, a few hun-
dred metres from what is now the Victoria & Albert (V&A) Waterfront.
Today this institution is a medical museum.[26]

After an interview before a board of five doctors, Christiaan went outside the office building and found a beautiful square, roughly the size
of a rugby field. Arranged around the sides of the square were half a
dozen barrack-like buildings, each housing patients with different infectious diseases such as tuberculosis, diphtheria, measles, scarlet fever and
meningitis. Christiaan wandered into one of the buildings and heard the
sound of crying children.

'It was no ordinary crying; this was the tragic sound of children who had been crying for a very long time.'

The building Christiaan had entered was where children were being treated for tuberculous meningitis (TB meningitis), one of the most extreme forms of TB in existence, then and now. It causes inflammation of the membranes that surround the brain and spinal cord. This can lead to extensive brain damage and is lethal.

'In those years TB meningitis was a common, serious and widespread disease,' writes Prof Lionel Opie, a former colleague of Barnard's.[27]

In the ward Christiaan encountered the steel cots that were designed to keep the young children inside – for their own safety. The babies displayed varying stages of abnormality due to the ravages of the dread disease.

'Some of the small bodies had heads as large as soccer balls. Never in my life had I seen such human suffering. The fact that they were young children magnified the suffering. The halls of hell must surely echo with the sounds these poor children were making,' Christiaan recalled.

The children's chances of survival were non-existent as there was no known cure.

'The children either died or were severely brain damaged by the illness. The only possible tiny hope was if the patients were treated at a very early stage in the disease. There was simply no effective treatment to save the children.'

The following day Christiaan was informed that he had the job. The new job included a perk: his family could move into the doctor's quarters above the matron's office at the hospital.[28]

He started working in the TB meningitis hall.

'I immediately started looking for answers, some solution to the nightmare of their agony. I began by researching the causes of the disease.'

TB occurs when tuberculosis bacteria are inhaled by a child, most often from an older family member with TB. The bacteria make their way to the child's lungs. Children suffering from malnutrition generally do not have the strength to fight these bacteria so they spread to the blood and elsewhere in the body. In some cases, the bacteria settle in the membrane around the brain and cause TB meningitis. Once this occurs, it is too late to do anything. The inflammation triggers the release of a protein, which settles on the base of the brainstem. This sediment blocks the usual draining of cerebral fluid from the brain into the body via the spinal cord.

'As a result of this blockage, the brain starts to suffer because of the fluid build-up. The brain starts to swell and this eventually leads to the head starting to swell. It changes the children into grotesque monsters.'[29]

Christiaan was desperate to alleviate the children's suffering. He believed that the answer lay in finding a way to stop the inflammation before the protein could be released.

The work was exhausting and lonely and done under terribly trying conditions. Christiaan had to work in untested territory with very little to go on. Often the young doctor would have to perform up to 40 painful lumbar punctures per day on his tiny patients. He worked until late at night, doing post-mortem investigations on the bodies of children he had tried to save only hours before. His goal was to develop new treatments for the illness but, despite his best efforts, the patients kept dying.

'The work done was experimental because there was no solution. The methods used had not been applied before and the risk was great.'[30]

One experimental treatment after another was tried without much success. The risk was acceptable only because the patients were already dying, and often horribly.

During this period Christiaan's views about apartheid's segregationist policies also became evident. He made it clear that he was opposed to the laws that determined coloured nurses could not be in charge of wards. He stated that the best nurses had to be in charge, regardless of skin colour.[31]

Christiaan's search for answers and better treatments started distinguishing him from his peers, as well as his older colleagues. While most accepted that the children would be brain damaged and die from the protein sediment, Christiaan worked tirelessly to find ways to alleviate the problem – if not to resolve it entirely.[32]

Eventually Christiaan completed a study of 259 cases of tuberculous meningitis over a two-year period between March 1951 and March 1953. It was to be the largest single clinical study ever undertaken into this disease.[33]

Christiaan's work did lead to better and improved treatment for the patients for whom there had been no hope at all. Prof Opie was one of the few who recalls Barnard's early work and his demeanour towards his desperately ill, mostly black and coloured, patients.

'His warmth and friendliness towards his young patients, often handicapped and disfigured, was evident. A person who could develop such relationships with such young patients could do so only through love and devotion to them.'[34]

On a personal level, Christiaan's long hours put huge pressure on his family life. This was exacerbated by the fact that he was in constant and intimate contact with young and attractive nurses, who may have been a necessary distraction in the terrible conditions in which he worked. The temptations were evidently too much for the young doctor at times, despite his family residing on the same premises as the hospital staff. There are many rumours of illicit affairs with female staff at the hospital in those early days. One was described as a 'nurse in the TB ward; a tall, blonde, blue-eyed woman with the body of an athlete and the grace of a model'.[35]

Christiaan couldn't hide all the evidence of his after-hours activities. One day, Louwtjie came across a letter that indicated an affair between her husband and one of the nurses.

'She wrote about how she met up with him at night when he was on night duty and how lonely her life had become since she had left the hospital. My world collapsed around me. I was 27 years old with two small children, 17 months and 6 months old. When I confronted Chris, he convinced me the nurse was crazy and was making the stories up.'[36]

Louwtjie believed him.

'There is no other man on earth who has the ability to mesmerise a woman like Chris can.'[37]

Christiaan's research into tuberculous meningitis formed the basis of his PHD thesis in medicine. In 1953, at the age of 31 years, he received his first doctorate.[38]

At the end of his two years at the City Hospital, Christiaan returned to Groote Schuur, determined to become a surgeon.[39]

Intestinal atresia

When he arrived back at Groote Schuur, Christiaan embarked on his next research project – the causes of intestinal atresia, which caused the deaths of thousands of babies shortly after birth. This condition is a life-threatening birth defect where there is a narrowing or absence of a portion of the intestine.

In the 1950s, doctors across the world did not know what caused this abnormality or how to treat it successfully. Often the only treatment was to remove sections of the underdeveloped intestine and reconnect the healthy segments, but this was successful only on the rare occasion.

Jannie Louw, head of surgery at Groote Schuur, had a long history of trying to deal with intestinal atresia. Soon after Christiaan's arrival at the hospital, Louw lost another young patient to this condition and asked Christiaan if he wanted to investigate the problem. He explained that he had a hunch that the birth defect was caused by the inhibition of blood flow to the intestine while the baby was in utero. But how could they prove such a theory?

Christiaan agreed to investigate and developed an experimental programme to test Louw's theory, using dogs as the subjects of the experiments. Marius Barnard later described his brother's research as 'fantastic'.[40]

'Chris would take pregnant dogs and place them under anaesthetic. Then he would remove a puppy from the womb, open the puppy's stomach and identify the small intestine. He would then tie off blood vessels to the pup's intestine before placing the puppy back inside the mother's womb. Ideally, the mothers would then give birth as usual. Then the puppies with their stitches were examined. As soon as their intestines were examined, the impact of the restricted blood flow could be seen.'[41]

However, these experiments were easier said than done. Most of the pregnant dogs aborted and some ate their pups after birth. For nine months Christiaan persisted with these experiments. He operated on 42 pregnant dogs, without success.[42]

And then, on the 43rd attempt, success! His efforts paid off and a dog gave birth to a pup with the black stitches clearly visible and it exhibited all the signs of an underdeveloped intestine.

Christiaan went further and developed a treatment for intestinal atresia based on this ground-breaking research. The treatment involved cutting out not only the affected sections of the intestine but also an additional section at each end. The research showed that the damage caused by the restricted blood flow affected the nerves in the area and therefore a much larger section of the intestine – 15 to 20 centimetres – had to be removed.

This research subsequently saved the lives of thousands of babies as the treatment was taken up internationally following the publication of the research.[43]

'The research led to a change in the treatment of the condition. Before the mortality rate had been 90%. Christiaan's research into intestinal atresia swung the mortality rate around to a 90% success rate,' Louw said.

He also lauded Barnard's ground-breaking work on babies in the womb.

'This opened up the way for surgeons who wanted to operate on human babies while they were in the womb.'

'Research is exciting,' Christiaan would tell a class of students some time later. 'It is like a detective novel. You search for the criminal by following the clues. Then you go forward and put it all together. Even the failures are interesting.'[44]

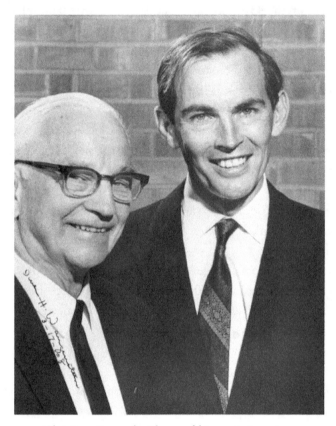

Christiaan Barnard with one of his greatest mentors,
Owen Wangensteen from the University of Minnesota.

CHAPTER 3

America

IN THE 1950S, THE AMERICAN UNIVERSITY OF MINNESOTA WAS THE SILICON Valley of cardiology. The university produced a spectacular number of world-famous pioneers in cardiology who would change the world of medicine forever.

The university was building on the successes of a rich tradition of innovation and progress that American surgeons had managed to achieve in the field of heart surgery. This progress had its roots in the battle-fields of the Second World War, proving the ancient Greek philosopher Hippocrates' point: 'He who wishes to be a surgeon must go to war.'

An American, Dr Michael DeBakey, one of the biggest pioneers in cardio-vascular surgery, once explained that before the war there wasn't much that could be done for patients with serious heart disease.

'It was all up to God.'

The American doctors who would change the course of cardiac sur-gery in the 1950s and 1960s all played a role during the Second World War. This devastating war, with its terrible new weaponry and tactics, led to an incredible flood of injuries, which placed doctors under immense pressure. This situation often forced doctors to think outside the box to try and save lives.

Initially surgeons prioritised less severely injured soldiers in an attempt to try and save as many lives as possible. More seriously injured soldiers were often merely given pain relief such as morphine, and sent to a hos-pice, to free up resources for those who were saveable. In the case of serious chest wounds, soldiers were generally made comfortable until they inevitably died. Medical science had not yet reached a stage where shrapnel could be removed safely from the chests of those who had managed to survive the original trauma.[1] Doctors had their hands full with patients who stood an actual chance of survival.

Dwight Harken

D-Day, 1944. Special hospitals were rolled out to treat the injured following the greatest invasion ever of the European mainland.[2]

This is where Dwight Harken enters the picture. Harken was part of the American Army's Medical Corps and would be the first man who dared to operate on human hearts on a large scale.[3] He was the Director of the 15th Heart Centre in Cirencester, England (an estimated 150 kilometres west of London), a hospital where patients with serious chest wounds were sent – patients who had very little hope of survival. Many of these soldiers had bits of shrapnel deep in their chests and some even had bullets in their hearts.[4]

The extent of the problem drove Dr Harken to start experimenting with surgery on the human heart. He understood that the bits of metal could not stay in the soldiers' chests. While it was life threatening to try and remove the shrapnel, it was worse to leave it inside the body.[5] The patient would die of sepsis or embolism.[6]

In the first place, if pieces of shrapnel are simply left in place, they create blood clots, which can shoot to the brain or other organs, causing a stroke or death. In the second place, bacteria form on the pieces of metal, leading to an infection known as bacterial endocarditis, a fatal disease that can now be cured with penicillin.[7]

Before the war Harken had been experimenting on dogs at Harvard University in Boston to determine if heart surgery was possible. His research involved inserting needles into dogs' hearts, and then removing the needles and trying to heal the animals. On a more practical level, he was trying to see if he could cut into a living heart, remove a piece of metal and keep the dog alive during and after the procedure.[8]

'What does a person require to get a licence to try something that has never been done before? First, a diagnosis that is absolute, second a condition that is incurable and finally, if there is any rational understanding of how to attack it, one has the right to try,' Harken said in an interview in the 1970s.[9]

As Harken was experimenting on the hearts of dogs in Boston, the war broke out and he was deployed to England. As fortune would have it, there he was confronted with young soldiers who had bits of metal inside their chests and their hearts. Harken wanted to do something for these young men.

On D-Day, 6 June 1944, a soldier was brought to Harken with a gaping chest wound. Shrapnel had penetrated the right side of his heart chamber. Harken was reminded of Rehn's reported method of 'the finger in the dam wall' and went into action.

In a later letter to his wife, he wrote: 'Suddenly, like a champagne cork, the bit of metal popped out and blood spurted like a fountain. I pressed my finger on it and applied stitches, closing the wound.'[10]

The operation was a success and Harken continued performing the procedure. By the end of the war, Harken had performed similar operations on 134 soldiers, removing bits of metal and bullets from chests. This included 19 bits of metal, which he removed directly from soldiers' hearts.

Harken wrote that there was always an incredible amount of blood loss during these operations and, accordingly, rapid and massive blood transfusions were necessary to keep the patients alive.

'Complete blood transfusions were done under immense pressure and at a rate of 1.5 litres per minute.'[11]

Remarkably, every single one of Harken's patients survived.[12]

'We discovered the heart was actually not such a mysterious and untouchable thing after all.'[13]

After the war, there were efforts to further Harken's work, with the aim of fixing defective heart valves. The challenge in those early years of the 1950s was that open-heart surgery was still impossible because the necessary technology simply did not exist. This forced doctors to stick to the established procedures of closed-heart surgery for heart-valve repairs (where the heart itself is not stopped or opened up), a difficult procedure with low success rates. While there were successes, many patients did not survive these procedures.

The basic procedures were improved gradually over time.[14]

Open-heart surgery

While these closed-heart procedures were a big step forward, there was still not much to be done for patients with more serious heart conditions. Open-heart surgery remained an impossibility.

The big challenge was blood circulation. Surgeons couldn't operate on the human heart without patients bleeding to death. One early experiment involved stopping the circulation of blood entirely but this gave surgeons only a small window of about four minutes before brain damage occurred due to lack of blood to the brain.

The next step in the evolution of heart surgery was taken by a Canadian, Bill Bigelow. Bigelow was inspired by ice fishermen and hibernating animals. He understood that hibernating animals' hearts beat much slower at lower temperatures so he started experimenting on humans under lowered body temperatures.[15]

Bigelow showed that by lowering the body's temperature, surgeons would have a much longer period in which to operate as the heart beats much slower. This idea increased operation times from 4 minutes to between 10 and 14 minutes.[16]

On 2 September 1952, two American surgeons from the University of Minnesota, Walton Lillehei and his friend and colleague John Lewis, performed the world's first open-heart surgery. The patient was a 5-year-old girl named Jackie Johnson, who was born with a life-threatening hole in her heart.[17] Patients with this affliction often developed severe infections and didn't survive long.

Before 1952, there had been no treatment available because of the blood-circulation challenge, which made it impossible for surgeons to work within the human heart for any length of time.[18]

It took the operating team 19 hours to cool Jackie's body temperature to 17 degrees. They did this by wrapping her in rubber blankets which conducted cold water. The medical team cut off her blood supply for five-and-a-half minutes while they fixed the hole in her heart.[19] The operation was a huge success and 11 days later Jackie was released from hospital.

In 1987, on the 35th anniversary of the surgery, Lillehei stood next to his former patient, who was still alive.

'She began a new era,' Lillehei said.[20]

Cross circulation and heart-lung machines

The cold treatment of patients was a huge success for smaller heart operations but still there was not much to be done for more serious heart ailments, which required more than 10 minutes of surgery.

Surgeons then tried to tackle this problem with a procedure called cross circulation. This amounted to connecting the blood circulation system of a patient to that of another – normally a parent. While surgeons worked on the patient, blood was circulated through the patient via the other person's body, which provided the necessary oxygenated blood.

'This was, in effect, an operation with a 200% mortality risk. Both parent and patient were at risk of dying,' explains heart surgeon David Cooper in his book Open Heart.[21]

Once again, Lillehei was the leader of the pack. On 26 March 1954, he successfully led a team in this procedure in which they managed to fix a highly complex ventricular heart-valve problem.

Lillehei and his team did 44 more cross-circulation procedures and 32 of the patients survived. In 28 cases the patients were young children whose parents acted as human heart-lung machines.[22] These children all had heart defects which could not be fixed using any other technique at that time.

It was thanks to the courageous efforts of Lillehei, who kept pushing the boundaries with new procedures, that many breakthroughs were made in those early days. He is justifiably considered the father of open-heart surgery.

However, the 200% mortality risk was not acceptable across the rest of the world and soon the proceedure was stopped. What became abundantly clear was that what was needed was a machine that could oxygenate blood and then pump that blood through a patient's body while they were under anaesthetic.

The result was the heart-lung machine, which could fulfil the functions of a patient's heart and lungs for hours by diverting the blood flow from the body to the machine and back through the body.[23]

The early pioneer of this machine was another American, John Gibbon.[24] By 1953 Gibbon had already used an early prototype of a heart-lung machine in a successful operation. He became disillusioned, however, by later failures.

After Gibbon's pioneering work, other hospitals, including the Mayo Clinic, and Lillehei and his colleague Richard de Wall, took the concept further and improved on it. Their improved model was the De Wall-Lillehei Pump Oxygenator developed at the University of Minnesota. Further improvements to Gibbon's machine led to the world's first commercial heart-lung machine, the Mayo-Gibbon machine, in 1958.[25] These machines made longer, more complex heart-surgery procedures possible.

Although the pioneering work done in the 1950s led to enormous progress in cardiology and cardiac surgery, there was still little that could be done for patients with severe heart damage. The only possible solution for these patients was a new heart but this would mean heart transplantation. But was something like this even possible?

Going to America

By 1956, Christiaan Barnard was a hard-working registrar and researcher at Groote Schuur Hospital, far removed from Minnesota.

By this time, he had completed a master's degree in internal medicine based on his work on intestinal atresia and was working towards becoming a surgeon.

However, his life changed the day he walked to his car in the parking lot at Groote Schuur and bumped into John Brock, the head of medicine at Groote Schuur. Brock had been contacted by Owen Wangensteen, the head of surgery at the University of Minnesota, under whom the university had become such a hotbed of surgical innovation. Wangensteen had been so impressed by the work of another South African doctor, Alan Thal, that he contacted Brock to find out if there were any other South African doctors who were of similar calibre.

There was one candidate: Christiaan Barnard.

That day in the parking lot, Brock asked, 'Chris, would you like to go to Minneapolis?'

'Minneapolis?'

'Yes, I can arrange a bursary with Prof Wangensteen.'

Christiaan knew the name: Wangensteen was famous for his pioneering work in surgery and was considered to be the best medical teacher in the world. The opportunity was immense. In Minnesota, there was also Walton Lillehei, who was doing spectacular work in open-heart surgery.[26]

Although Christiaan knew hardly anything about Minneapolis – he initially confused it with Indianapolis – the answer was a simple one.

'Yes, I would like that very much.'[27]

Barnard received a Dazian Foundation bursary, which would enable him to pursue further studies in the United States.[28] But by this stage the Barnards were in deep financial trouble. The small salary paid to state doctors gave them few options. With Christiaan returning to full-time studies, the family, with two young children, would have even less income. There was no alternative: Christiaan would have to go to America alone, while Louwtjie would remain in Cape Town and be the family's breadwinner. She had a job as a nurse in the Stuttafords store in Adderley Street. Louwtjie and the children would join Christiaan in Minnesota at a later stage.[29]

In December 1955, at the age of 33, Christiaan Barnard flew to

Minneapolis, a world far removed from anything he knew.[30]

From a medical point of view, Christiaan's timing was perfect. He arrived in Minneapolis just as the field of open-heart surgery was exploding, thanks to new technology, which included the heart-lung machine. Although he initially went to America with the intention of specialising in general surgery – following on his success with intestinal atresia, which had made waves worldwide. Christiaan spent the first eight months in the animal laboratory where he worked on new techniques involving general surgery to the throat and the small intestine. Then the heart-lung machine changed his course and refocused him on cardiac surgery.[31]

'By chance I walked past a laboratory one day where Vince Gott was experimenting with a heart-lung machine.'[32]

Gott was managing Lillehei's laboratory and asked Barnard to lend a hand with the machine during an operation. This was the turning point. Barnard discovered his new obsession and soon after this he moved to work under Lillehei, with Wangensteen's permission.

Things were not easy for the Karoo boy. His finances were so bad that he had to resort to mowing lawns and shovelling snow for money to buy food. There was very little time for making new friends or relaxing.

'A person learns a lot doing things like that. One thing I discovered was that one cannot make money shovelling snow.'[33]

Christiaan eventually spent more than two years in Minneapolis, from 1 January 1956 to 30 June 1958.[34]

'In those two-and-a-half years he managed to do what usually took five to six years,' Lillehei later remarked. 'He completed a house doctorship in general surgery and cardiothoracic surgery. At the same time, he spent half his time, if not more, in the experimental laboratory. He was an excellent researcher and very productive. His fellow registrars at the time included Vincent Gott and Norman Shumway. But Chris Barnard stood out in this group. I think one of the reasons was his intense ability to work very hard. He was also very intelligent.'[35]

This was quite a statement from a revered man in the field of cardiac surgery, considering that the best cardiac-surgery brains in the world were in Minneapolis.

Lillehei also recalled how Barnard had the ability to be extremely charming on the one hand but, on the other, he could provoke intense dislike 'because he was always so unconventional and outspoken'.[36]

Personal troubles

Six months after Christiaan left South Africa, his family joined him in the United States. The journey was a harrowing one for Louwtjie, who had to travel by herself with two young children in tow. Matters were exacerbated when Christiaan, due to his huge workload, was not there to meet them in Boston, as arranged. Instead, the exhausted Louwtjie had to find her own way to Minneapolis, a daunting task for a country girl from South Africa with limited funds and two small children.[37] This increased the tension between the Barnards.

In addition, Christiaan had been having affairs with at least two other women in the time he had been in the States. One was a Swedish nurse, Trudy Nordstrom. Christiaan never told her that he was married, with two children, and she left him when she eventually found out.

By the time Louwtjie was on her way to join him, Christiaan had embarked on a second affair, with a 20-year-old student named Sharon Jorgenson, who worked in the surgery department in her spare time.[38] Louwtjie was unaware of these affairs.

Despite his unfaithfulness, Christiaan worked desperately hard to prepare a home for his family, notwithstanding his financial challenges. Unfortunately, Louwtjie – the Namibian farm girl – struggled to adapt to life in Minnesota.[39]

John Perry, one of Christiaan's friends in those days, said, 'I think the children enjoyed living in America, but Louwtjie was very homesick and unhappy from the start. She had few friends and Chris was busy at the hospital day and night.'[40]

While in America, Christiaan laid the foundation for his future, but he also received the worst news any potential surgeon could receive.

Deirdre Barnard recalls, 'The first indication that something was seriously wrong, happened on one of those innocent days – as often is the case with things that change your life forever. We went on a family outing to the ice-skating rink. It was nice to do something together as a family, where my parents were laughing together and encouraging us. Those were some of the happiest times. Ice-skating is a cold business. We all got cold, especially our feet. But my father experienced the cold as a deep and continuous pain that didn't want to go away.'[41]

At that time Christiaan was spending hours each day standing around operating tables and initially he blamed the pain in his feet on the ice-skates he had borrowed from his friend John Perry.

'The shoes had been narrow and squeezing my feet. The next morning my right foot was very sore. Colleagues said it was possibly a small fracture. But then my foot started swelling up and then my hands started getting sore,' Christiaan noted later.[42]

'Eventually my other joints were also painful so I went to see a specialist. He did a thorough consultation and took blood tests to confirm the diagnosis. Then with great empathy he shared the news I had been dreading. I was suffering from rheumatoid arthritis.'[43]

Christiaan was only 34 years old when he received this diagnosis.

'It was an affliction that attacked my most precious asset – my hands.'

This situation taught the young Christiaan a valuable lesson – the importance of giving patients some hope.

'I was a young, aspiring surgeon, rapidly learning all there was to know about all the intricacies of open-heart surgery. All surgeries are physically and mentally challenging; one often has to stand for long hours performing delicate procedures. To perform in a challenging surgical environment when it is necessary to work at maximum efficiency, it is difficult if your body starts contracting with pain and the joints in your hands are swollen and sore.'[44]

Rheumatoid arthritis is incurable and, as a doctor, Christiaan fully understood the implications. The specialist who treated him was at the Mayo Clinic, close to the University of Minnesota.

'The consultant who delivered my diagnosis, however, said I would not become crippled. That saved me. Initially I couldn't help but think of that old lady in my fourth year at UCT. My first thoughts were, "Here I am, a young man trying to be a surgeon, and with hands like those that would be completely impossible".'[45]

The diagnosis led to much soul searching.

'Despite my arthritis I kept working hard, so hard I set a record in gaining my master's and doctorate degrees from the University of Minnesota in a short period. At the same time, I was starting to do open-heart surgeries. Often I'd put in 18-hour days, many spent on my feet in theatre. In some way, I managed to handle the intense stress and long hours.'[46]

Deirdre says her father was very lucky, 'not because of the painful and paralysing disease he had received but rather the positive and hopeful manner in which the doctor who delivered the diagnosis, spoke to him. That doctor discussed the various forms of rheumatoid arthritis and explained that while the diagnosis could not be wished away, there was some positive news. While the disease would affect him, the specific strain that my father was diagnosed with, would not lead to him ending in a wheelchair, stripped of all quality of life. He gave my father hope. "Nothing is more important than that," my father said later.'[47]

Throughout his career, this was a sentiment that Barnard would apply to his own patients. Despite the severity of the diagnosis, there was always a chance that matters could improve. To give up on hope made no sense.

'My father would see the possibilities in the most devastating medical prognosis and was always positive about life even though his arthritis and, later, his asthma would afflict him for the rest of his life. The disease became his constant companion [from] the day it was diagnosed in Minneapolis.'[48]

Louwtjie and the two children spent a year in the United States and then returned to Cape Town to wait for Christiaan to complete his studies.

Back to Cape Town

Professionally, Barnard's time in Minnesota was a giant success. It laid the foundation for his future and gave him the opportunity to learn from and work with the pioneers and leaders in cardiac surgery – the very best.

Barnard was granted a Master of Science degree and a PhD within two years and nine months – a University of Minnesota record.[49] He also spent invaluable hours working under top heart surgeons such as Richard Varco and Lillehei, where he learnt about open-heart surgery and the techniques to repair many heart defects, including the ones afflicting many children, and gained expertise with the heart-lung machine.[50]

'I was lucky. They were busy with work that grabbed my imagination. Open-heart surgery in those days was a giant leap forward in medicine.'[51]

Wangensteen, the head of Department, was amazed at the South African's ability to work hard and he desperately tried to keep Barnard in America. Later, Wangensteen would say that, out of all the doctors who had passed through his hands in Minnesota, including great trail-blazers like Lillehei and Norman Shumway, Christiaan Barnard was the best registrar he'd seen.

Wangensteen wrote long letters to Jannie Louw asking to keep Barnard for longer, but Louw was adamant that he wanted him back. Christiaan swung the decision in Louw's favour as he was determined to return to Cape Town.

When he completed his term at the University of Minnesota, the American National Health Institute gave Barnard a gift of a De Wall-Lillehei heart-lung machine and funding of US$6 000 to assist him with his work in Cape Town. This gift was made possible thanks to the intervention of Wangensteen, who made a few phone calls to Washington.[52]

In correspondence with the Commonwealth Fund in New York in November 1957, Wangensteen wrote: 'I'm writing to hear if you would consider making a donation of vital equipment and funding for a year for Dr Barnard. I have a feeling it will be an investment that will pay off in a big way.'[53]

On a personal level, the time in America was disastrous for the Barnards. Christiaan's relationship with Louwtjie was in trouble, with the dark clouds of his affairs adding to the drama.

Barnard left Sharon Jorgenson behind with a heavy heart.

'I had to tear myself away from a girl I had fallen in love with. As a married man, I should have known better but for more than a year Sharon was very dear to my heart. When I left she begged me not to leave but my sense of responsibility tore me away from her.'[54]

In addition, Barnard's diagnosed rheumatoid arthritis was a hammer blow, landed at a time when he was trying to establish himself as a cardiac surgeon.

Two-and-a-half years after had he left Cape Town, Christiaan Barnard finally arrived home. In 1958, he joined the staff of Groote Schuur Hospital as a cardiologist and Director of Surgical Research.

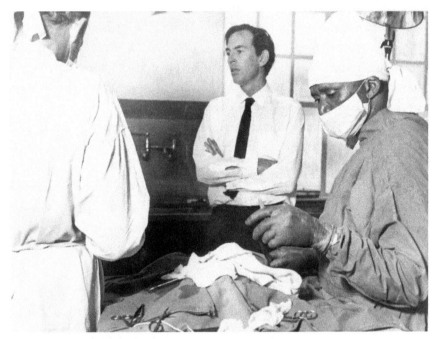

*Christiaan Barnard in the animal laboratory at UCT. To his left is
Hamilton Naki. Naki was one of a team of assistants who helped the
surgeons with their experimentation.*

CHAPTER 4

The assistants

THE JS MARAIS RESEARCH LABORATORY AT UCT STARTED OUT AS NOTH-
ing more than two rooms in the pathology museum building, which
were given to the Cardiology Department out of frustration rather than
magnanimity.

In the 1950s, this laboratory was stocked with animals, mostly dogs,
baboons and rats. These were used in medical experiments to assist surgeons and other specialists in preparatory work before big operations.
Inside this innocuous-looking building, surgical techniques were tested,
honed and improved.[1]

This laboratory often got unsolicited support from the State
Veterinarian for experimental work. For instance, once it received an
offer of 24 mules at a cost of R4 each, but this had to be politely turned
down because of space constraints.[2]

While most of the experimental work was done on dogs, baboons were
often preferred for experimental surgery because their blood types were
compatible with those of humans. In addition, baboons were abundant
in the province and because they were classified as vermin, they were not
too hard to get hold of.[3]

As Groote Schuur was a state hospital, budgetary constraints were
always a headache. These small budgets meant that there was always a
shortage of support staff. In the early years of the laboratory and experimental research at UCT, one of the pioneering researchers, Robert Goetz,
started pulling in cleaners and general workers from around the university and training them to assist him in the laboratory with the animal

experiments.[4] By 1958 Goetz had left the country, and the research facility was falling into disuse. Then Barnard returned.

Nine months before Barnard returned from Minnesota, another Groote Schuur surgeon had attempted open-heart surgery using an early prototype of a heart-lung machine. The surgeon had had little previous experience on the machine and the operation was catastrophic, with the patient bleeding to death.[5]

This disastrous experience resulted in Louw, the head of surgery at Groote Schuur, placing a moratorium on all open-heart operations until Barnard's return. He knew that Christiaan had received a heart-lung machine. Louw never doubted that Barnard would return and his trust was not in vain.

Upon Barnard's return, he – together with Louw – decided to establish a new open-heart surgical team that would work with the heart-lung machine. This team would be based in the research laboratory, which Barnard took charge of.

The heart-lung machine, which Wangensteen had arranged for his star pupil, arrived in Cape Town two weeks after Barnard. He drove to the Cape Town docks to personally take possession of the precious machine, which he transported back to Groote Schuur in his car.

'I wasn't prepared to trust anyone else with the job. I had taken great care in packing and shipping the machine in America and had fussed over it all through customs.'[6]

'Chrisjan,' he could hear his father say, 'if you want something done right, do it yourself.'

By the time the machine arrived, the team had already formed. Besides Barnard, the initial open-heart surgery team consisted of a technician, Carl Goosen, a surgical assistant, Dr Malcolm 'Mac' McKenzie, and a coloured assistant named Victor Pick, known as Big Vic.[7] Big Vic already had 18 years' service in the laboratory and had been the senior laboratory assistant for a number of these.[8] Initially he had been employed as a cleaner and dishwasher, then as an assistant under Goetz.[9]

Together these four men unpacked the first heart-lung machine in Africa and started putting it together in the research laboratory, with

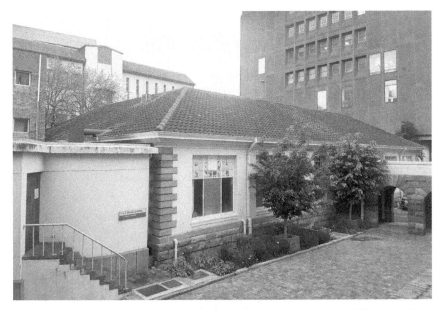

In the foreground is the JS Marais research facility as it appears today. This was where
Chris Barnard performed his first reported animal heart transplant in 1963. The tall
dark building at the back is the Chris Barnard building. It houses the Chris Barnard
Division of Cardiothoracic Surgery at UCT.

© JAMES-BRENT STYAN

other colleagues popping in every now and then to have a look at 'Chris's machine'.[10] Barnard described the machine as a dozen different sciences that were thrown together into one unit meant to replace the heart and lungs of a person. If it worked properly.

'If it didn't work properly, the machine was an instrument of death. Each component had a purpose to keep a patient alive, but each component had the potential to kill too.'[11]

Barnard later stated that the De Wall-Lillehei Oxygenator – which is part of the Heart of Cape Town museum exhibit today – took the team to a place that had been impossible till then: the inside of the human heart.

'It made open-heart surgeries possible and would eventually bring the heart transplant within reach.'[12]

Husband and wife

On his return from America, all was not well on the home front. Christiaan had last seen his family 14 months earlier. During this time, his letters had become less and less frequent, to the extent that he would write to them only once a month and sometimes even less often. Louwtjie recalls that his letters gradually became more like 'notes from the pen of a stranger and were increasingly cold'.[13]

By the time he landed at Cape Town's DF Malan International Airport, Louwtjie, too, was convinced there had to be another woman.

'But I still loved him. The first two days following his return were a charade. And then he left on a three-day hunting trip to Ceres. A few days later, the children and I also went there to visit our mutual friends where Chris was staying. Eventually the children remained behind when Chris and I drove back to Cape Town. In silence. When we got home I said we had to talk openly.'

'About what?'

'Your strange behaviour and the woman in Minneapolis.'

'I don't know what you're talking about.'

Barnard had all sorts of excuses.

Louwtjie kept pressing until he eventually conceded she was correct. Christiaan was in love with another woman in Minneapolis.

'She's wonderful. You cannot expect me to turn my love on and off like a tap. I will love her like I want to and, at the moment, there's nothing you can do about it,' Barnard stated defiantly.

Louwtjie felt faint.

'Suddenly my whole world was a desert. I didn't want to believe Chris had scorned me for another woman. How could he still sleep with me and win me over with his sweet talking yet coldheartedly admit he loved another woman? I simply couldn't accept that this man had replaced me with another woman. The children made things difficult. They were so happy to see their father; how could I make it a once per week thing? It was not easy. Things were often so bad; I even left him for two weeks at one stage.'[14]

48

The turning point was the death of Adam Barnard. After his retirement, Adam and Maria had settled in Prince Albert for a while, but he had been diagnosed with cancer and his health had deteriorated. Adam's final wish was to be closer to his beloved forest, so he and Maria sold all they had and returned to Knysna.[15]

In the weeks before his father died, Christiaan went to great trouble to have him treated in Cape Town. But it was for nought because there was nothing more to be done for him. Adam returned to Knysna, where he died with Maria at his side.

'Of all the days in the year, Father chose to die on my birthday,' Johannes Barnard recalled.[16]

None of Adam's four sons managed to reach him before he died. Maria later told her sons that Adam's last words on his deathbed were, 'Where are our children?'[17]

'[Adam] was a wonderful man and father-in-law. The children called him *oupatjie*. He was small in stature but great in spirit. He never forced his faith and religion on others, including his sons and instead chose to make his life a living example of living out his faith daily. He was the embodiment of what he preached,' Louwtjie recalls.[18]

Adam was 84 when he died. His funeral was attended by hundreds of members of the coloured community whom he had served, and who been part of his life over the years. Many had travelled the 300 kilometres from Beaufort West to Knysna to be there and they carried *oupatjie*'s coffin on their shoulders to his grave.

'It looked like the coffin was floating above us. The people for whom my father had lived were now carrying him to his grave. They were silent. Their faces filled with grief. They carried him as if he was a part of them. Too many hands and shoulders to count. Each one carried the coffin as if it was a far heavier load than just the old, tiny man inside. They were carrying a part of themselves to the grave – and their own sorrow went along with them,' wrote Chris.[19]

Marius Barnard and his family were living in Salisbury (today Harare) at the time and couldn't make it to Adam's funeral. His wife, Inéz, had also just given birth to their third child, a boy.

'We had been struggling to come up with a name, but when Marius was so heartbroken, the decision was easy. I told him our son's name would be Adam,' Inéz recounts.

The death of Adam Barnard was a great loss but it brought Louwtjie and Chris together again, perhaps poetically the old man's last gift to his family.

'Chris needed me and I could help him and so we came together again. Our existence became calm and normal again,' said Louwtjie.[20]

About a year after he first returned to Cape Town, Christiaan went overseas again to attend medical conventions and returned to Minneapolis.

'While he was there he wrote me the most beautiful letter in which he apologised for everything and declared his love for me. The day of his return to Cape Town he had two dozen red roses sent to me. On the card was written: "Thank you, I will always love you, Chris."'[21]

The first open-heart surgery

They had to start from the bottom, working on a tiny budget. Often there was no specialised equipment and the team had to be inventive or make do with what they had. Goosen turned out to be a huge asset in this regard. He was exceptionally innovative and later went on to do brilliant work designing and building artificial heart valves alongside Barnard.[22] At Groote Schuur, the new team impressed Barnard from the start. The team had calibrated the machine and tested it thoroughly – initially on dogs. The first two dogs died due to technical complications. A further 24 times the machine was tested with increasing degrees of complexity but without any further complications. After the last tests, the team was ready to test the machine on a human patient.[23]

Finally, it was time to pick the first human patient for Groote Schuur's first open-heart surgery. Barnard had been cautioned by Lillehei to start with easier operations, thereby reducing the risk of failure and, accordingly, the pressure on the team.

'I decided that the first patient would be Joan Pick, a 15-year-old coloured girl with a pulmonary valve stenosis,' Barnard said.[24]

Joan Pick was Big Vic's niece. Before the operation she was a complete invalid because her narrowed heart valve affected the blood flow to her lungs.[25]

The operation in July 1958 wasn't expected to require much more than placing Joan Pick on the machine, opening up her heart, making three small incisions to the heart valve and then closing her up again and taking her off the machine.[26]

The operation, which started at 9.30am, turned out to be much more complicated than expected and eventually took seven-and-a-half hours.[27]

'The first operation was utterly stimulating but very stressful. I not only had to keep an eye on the heart-lung machine, I had to make sure it was working correctly. When my assistants and I started the operation, I helped them open the chest and put her on the machine. Then I went to help the technicians with the machine, after which I went back again to help the surgeons with the operation. Every time I had to pass through the disinfectant procedures,' Barnard recounts.[28]

After the operation, Barnard accompanied Joan Pick to the recovery ward. He was exhausted and hungry but refused all offers of food and water while he kept vigil at her bedside, monitoring her vital signs.[29] Joan awoke and the operation was declared a complete success. The success story made the front pages of all the local newspapers.

The *Cape Times* – which referred to the heart-lung machine as a 'robot heart' stated on 28 July 1958, 'The first successful open-heart surgery in Africa was performed by Groote Schuur Hospital on a 15-year-old Cape Coloured girl.'[30]

This was to be the start of great things for the cardiac surgery team from Groote Schuur Hospital.

Joan Pick went on to live another 42 years.[31]

The laboratory team

The experimental work done on the animals in the surgical research laboratory enabled the Barnard team to prepare for complex open-heart operations and organ transplantation.

The work was never easy. For instance, Barnard himself was bitten by a dog one day, which caused his arthritis to flare up. Still the team pressed on with the heart-lung machine at the centre of it all.

'It sounds like a bit of dry medical history,' Barnard wrote in later years with regard to the heart-lung machine, 'but it wasn't. It was blood, sweat and not a few tears.'

The team's work also provided new hope for many patients for whom there had previously been no chance.[32]

'We learnt as we went along. Techniques were tested in the laboratory and implemented in the theatre. When there were problems in theatre, they were investigated in the laboratory.'[33]

The laboratory team worked as a tight unit under the leadership of Pick. Along with Pick, the mainstays were Hamilton Naki, Prescott Madlingozi, John Rossouw and Frederick Snyders, nicknamed Boots.[34]

Madlingozi was a big man who had served in the Second World War as a soldier. He was fluent in German and French, abilities that proved to be extremely useful later when Groote Schuur had to communicate with the many foreigners who streamed in after the heart transplant.[35]

Madlingozi was also a star rugby player, playing hooker for teams that included the Leopards, a national representative side of the South African Rugby Board, which governed black rugby under apartheid. At the time, black players were not allowed to play for the Springbok side due to the segregationist laws of the country. Some sources state that Madlingozi was captain of the Leopards but this seems to be incorrect. The Springbok Rugby Experience Museum in Cape Town confirms that Madlingozi made his debut in the team considered to be the African Springboks in 1966.

'However, he wasn't the captain. The captain at that time was Norman Mbiko and after Mbiko it was Thomson Magxala. In those days, there were many black rugby players playing for the Leopards who were working at UCT,' says museum representative Hendrik Snyders.[36]

Each member of the laboratory team had unique skills: Boots was very good at anaesthetising baboons before the animals knew what was going on.[37] Big Vic ensured that the laboratory was ready before the experiments. Naki was another anaesthetist who specialised in liver and kidney work on dogs.

While these men were acknowledged in books after the first heart transplant, including in Barnard's autobiography, the media largely ignored them and the team were largely forgotten until matters took a turn after Naki's death in 2005.

Hamilton Naki

Naki was born in the town of Ngcingane in the Centane district in the old homeland area of the Transkei. He attended school until Standard 6 after which he left home for Cape Town in 1940 to look for work.[38] He got a job as a gardener at UCT.

Fourteen years later, he was transferred to the medical school where Prof Goetz, who was busy with cardiovascular research, ran into him. Goetz pulled Naki in to help in the laboratory as an assistant. Although Naki had no formal education, he would eventually do the work of an anaesthetist and prepare the animals for research experiments. He assisted Goetz with many interesting research projects, including determining how the giraffe's blood-circulatory system works.

Naki was efficient and competent in the work he was required to do. In later years, he could perform complex liver transplants on animals, experimental work that Barnard himself never did. Barnard was interested only in hearts.

'He had more skills than I did when it came to the technical things,' Barnard recalled later.

Naki was known to be a sharp dresser and his pride in his appearance was reflected in his work. He eventually completed 42 years of service at

UCT and provided guidance to thousands of aspirational young medical students who passed through the laboratory during the course of their studies.

When he died, Naki became world famous following the release of a controversial documentary film and several resultant obituaries from credible sources, including *The Economist* and *Time* magazine. These sources claimed that Naki had been let down by Barnard and the apartheid regime, and stated that he had actually played a crucial role during the first heart transplant at Groote Schuur. Some reports even indicated that Naki had removed the donor heart during the operation in 1967.

Nothing could be further from the truth.

Anwar Mall, an emeritus professor at UCT, had known Naki since 1981 when the two started working together.[39] He says there can be no doubt that Naki and his co-assistants in the laboratory played a significant role in the research being undertaken at UCT and that they were involved in the preparatory work for the heart-transplant programme.

'However, it is a fact that neither Naki nor any of the other assistants were present the night that Denise Darvall's heart was transplanted into the chest of Louis Washkansky.'

Besides the fact that Naki was black and apartheid legislation would have prevented him being present at the bed of a white patient, the fact is that Naki was simply not qualified to enter an operating theatre in any hospital. Mall says that there is no doubt that Naki was an extraordinary person and it is tragic that the world knows about the Barnards but not about Naki.

'Sadly, the image of Hamilton Naki was damaged by the misinformation that was spread after his death. I will repeat: he had no part in the first heart transplantation in 1967. He was never involved with human patients. It would have been illegal since he was not a qualified medical doctor. Naki never qualified as a doctor, but he received an honorary master's degree from UCT shortly before he died.'

On 9 June 2005, after Naki's death, obituaries in the *Guardian*, *The New York Times* and the other publications all carried incorrect data relating to Naki's role in 1967.[40]

This prompted the university to set the record straight and, in the process, Naki's role and contribution to research was tragically undermined.

'He wasn't just a colleague, he was a mentor and personal friend. We worked together under Prof Rosemary Hickman, another close colleague of Hamilton,' says Mall.

Mall remembers Naki as being religious and always arriving at work with a Bible tucked under his arm. 'He was a wonderful man who did a lot with regards to research and providing guidance to students who passed through the lab. But when it comes to the transplant, he had no role and, in fact, wasn't even aware it was happening. It happened over a weekend and there would have been no means to contact him. Hammy was a man with humble roots whose family was in the Transkei, so he was resident in a hostel in the township. Despite all that, he taught himself complex medical techniques without a formal education. Upon being asked how he knew what he did, he said he had stolen with his eyes.'

The Economist and other media, including medical journals such as *The Lancet* and the *British Medical Journal*, had to place corrections.

'We have since been assured by surgeons at Groote Schuur, the hospital where the transplant was performed, that Mr Naki was nowhere near the operating theatre. As a black, and as a person with no formal medical qualifications, he was not allowed to be. The surgeons who removed the donor's heart were Marius Barnard, Christiaan Barnard's brother, and Terry O'Donovan. A source close to Mr Naki once asked him where he was when he first heard about the transplant. He replied that he had heard of it on the radio. Later, he apparently changed his story.'

'He changed it, it seems, not simply because of the confusion of old age, but because of pressure from those around him,' *The Economist* stated in its correction.

'To report this misapprehension is doubly sad, apart from our own regret at being caught up in it. It is sad that the shadow of apartheid is still so long in South Africa that blacks and whites can tell the same narrative in quite different ways, each suspecting the motives of the other. And it is especially tragic that it should have involved Mr Naki, a man considered "wonderful" by both sides, black and white, and whose life should still be seen as an inspiration,' *The Economist* stated.[41]

Another surgeon to correct the narrative was John Terblanche. He had been Barnard's research assistant in the laboratory in 1960 and had assisted Barnard with transplanting dog hearts. He said that the falsehoods around Naki's role during the first heart transplant cast aspersions on the legacy of Naki, the Barnards and the entire transplantation team.[42] He said that Naki's role at the time consisted of acting as a nurse and helping with the animals rather than as a surgical assistant.[43] This would have included duties like applying anaesthesia.

Big Vic was still in charge in the laboratory at that time and continued in this role until 1969 when he died in a motor-vehicle accident.

'After Pick's tragic death, Naki's role as surgical assistant in the lab started. Therefore, to claim he was an integral part of the first heart-transplantation team and that he was involved with the first operation, is fiction,' said Terblanche.[44]

Hickman, the formidable surgeon who was in charge of the research lab from 1968 to 1995, corroborates these facts. She was appointed to this position in 1968 by Jannie Louw and was only the second female surgeon to be appointed at Groote Schuur. Naki and the rest of the team reported to her for years. She confirmed that Naki was an exceptional man.

'However, he had no part in the first heart transplant. Hammy only ever worked on animals. It's a great pity the falsehoods that are linked to him. There is no doubt however that the assistants in the animal laboratory only ever worked on animals and never had any human patients.'[45]

This should not detract from the important role these assistants played in the 1960s. Marius Barnard later said that the transplant team would not have exchanged these men 'for anything'.[46]

The respect was mutual. For example, Victor Pick named his youngest son Marius.

Peter Hawthorne, an ex-*Time* correspondent who wrote extensively about the men in the research laboratory in his book, *The Transplanted Heart*, published in 1968, recounts how Marius said, it was a 'great honour' and spoke with 'great emotion relating to these men'. Hawthorne wrote about how the Barnards had acknowledged the role of the laboratory assistants in 1968, when Marius described Naki as one of the best anaesthesiologists he had ever seen.

Marius Barnard did many open-heart surgeries on dogs with the help of Big Vic and Naki. Together they put artificial valves in dogs' hearts and their procedures were as good as any done elsewhere.

'Victor and Hammy would prepare everything and get the dogs ready for the open-heart operation. Hammy would apply anaesthesia and then I would place the dogs on bypass. Then Hammy would leave the anaesthesia and the two of them would help me during the operation,' Marius Barnard explained to Hawthorne.[47]

Hawthorne personally experienced the camaraderie between the Barnards and the team of assistants. 'With ease and confidence of experience they worked together with all the confidence of qualified surgeons and technicians.'

When Deirdre Barnard was in primary school in Rondebosch, her class paid a visit to the medical campus to see what her father was doing.

'He was very keen to show the schoolgirls the hospital,' Deirdre recalls.[48]

On the day of their visit the assistants had gone to great trouble to make things interesting.

'The bad side of things was that the things they showed us, the work they were busy with, led to many of the girls fainting. That day Boots helped all the young girls, who were fainting, so kind-heartedly. Boots and Hamilton were always such friendly and helpful people. I think Boots got his nickname from the big white boots he would always wear.'

The young Standard 3 pupils from Rustenburg Girls School were also saddened by the lot of the animals that were being used for research purposes.

When discussing animal research in an interview in 1978, Christiaan Barnard said that he loved animals too. 'I just love people more.'

There can be no doubt that Naki was a talented experimental surgeon. Sadly, he never had the opportunity to qualify as a doctor and treat people and there can be no doubt that he was not present at the first heart transplantation. The tragic reality of apartheid-era legislation simply made that impossible.

CHAPTER 5

The competition

IN A STRANGE TWIST TO THE TALE, CHRISTIAAN BARNARD DID NOT perform the first heart transplant on a human. This honour goes to an American named James Hardy. Hardy boasts the unique record of also having done the world's first lung transplantation.[1]

However, Hardy is best known for the heart transplant he performed on 68-year-old Boyd Rush on 23 January 1964. The difference between his operation and the world-famous one performed by Barnard in 1967 was that Hardy transplanted a chimpanzee's heart into Rush and the operation was unsuccessful.

Hardy was desperate to do something to prolong Rush's life, but there was no human heart available, so he decided to push ahead and use a chimpanzee's heart instead. The transplanted organ initially beat feebly, but eventually it was too small to make any meaningful difference. Rush never regained consciousness and died on the table 90 minutes after the transplantation.

Hardy's operation was still a remarkable breakthrough in many aspects but it never really got the attention from the medical fraternity that Barnard's would later get. Part of the problem was that Hardy was based at a hospital in Jackson in the southern state of Mississippi, a state at the time mostly in the news for its racial discrimination.[2]

In addition, Hardy's hospital bosses handled the information poorly, initially stating that Hardy had 'cut out the heart of a dead man, brought it back to life and then transplanted it'.[3] They were reportedly concerned about the possible fallout, were it to be made known that a chimpanzee's

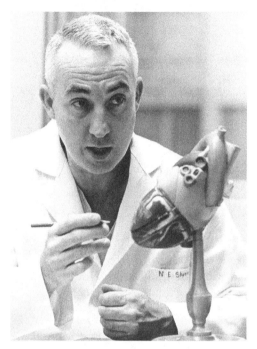

Norman Shumway from Stanford University in the USA, was one of the greatest pioneers in heart transplantation. Shumway was heavily favoured to be the surgeon who would perform the world's first heart transplant.

PHOTOGRAPH COURTESY OF THE STANFORD MEDICAL HISTORY CENTER.

heart had been used. Hardy was immediately painted as a ghoulish doctor. Then the hospital had to admit that an animal heart had been used and this exacerbated things.

A few days later Hardy appeared at a medical conference before a room full of his peers in New York. When he stood up to address the audience on his historic heart transplantation, the chairman of the meeting, Willem Kolff, made a snide racial remark for no reason.

'Do they keep blacks in one cage and chimpanzees in other cages in the Southern States?' he asked.[4]

Immediately the entire audience was against Hardy, who still had to go ahead with his presentation, which was not well received. Not a single person applauded him.[5] Later Kolff stated that he had made the comment as a joke.

The negative attention resulted in Hardy's withdrawal from the transplantation business. He decided to maintain a low profile, given that his hospital was dependent on funding from the National Institutes. Hardy did not want to risk losing funding as a result of negative press sentiment.[6]

Behind the Iron Curtain

There was another surgeon who had been experimenting with heart transplantation before Hardy, but his work was largely unknown due to other unique circumstances.

Vladimir Demikhov was a Russian working behind the Iron Curtain in Moscow. The first time the world heard about him was in 1954, when an audience of surgeons attending a conference of the Moscow Medical Fellowship saw a medical anomaly on the stage before them: a large white dog with two heads. Both heads were moving and the one tail was wagging.

In reality, this was one dog with the upper body of another attached to its neck. Still, the world heard about the two-headed dog, thanks to an article in *Time* that reported on the matter.

The dog experiment was the product of Demikhov, who was head of the transplantation laboratory at the Soviet Academy of Medical Science, which was established in 1944.[7] This was the top scientific and medical institution in the Soviet Union and was renamed the Russian Academy of Medical Sciences in 1992.

For years Demikhov had been doing experimental organ transplants on animals. In the 1940s and 1950s, he performed many first transplantations, including heart transplants on dogs. In 1946 and shortly thereafter, he performed a heart-lung transplant on a dog.[8]

The Iron Curtain and the limitations it placed on travel and freedom of speech served as a cruel inhibitor and Demikhov was largely unknown outside Russia for decades. In addition, poor record-keeping of Demikhov's work in those early days means that most of his work is still largely unverifiable. *The New York Times* obituary on Demikhov states that the Russian did pioneering work in organ transplantation.[9]

Demikhov was undoubtedly one of the world's greatest experimental surgeons. What is even more remarkable is the fact that he did most of his transplants without the use of heart-lung machines or hypothermia. Instead, he relied largely on his surgical speed and his self-designed system of organ preservation during operations.[10]

Despite his dog heart transplantation in 1946, he is known mostly for his head transplantation. Many films and books from the Cold War era reference the doctor from the Soviet Union, who is often depicted as an evil, experimental, ghoulish individual – undoubtedly part of the Cold War propaganda at the time.

Demikhov's international isolation only ensured that speculation and myths relating to his work and abilities abounded. His head transplant in 1954 raised eyebrows around the world and there was debate, even in his own country, about the morality and ethics of the work he was doing.[11]

Once, in the 1950s, a committee from the Russian Ministry of Health decided that Demikhov's work was unethical and he was ordered to desist from doing experimental work. However, his boss was the Surgeon General of the Soviet Armed Forces and he had sufficient authority and independence to allow Demikhov to ignore the Ministry.

The Russian's isolation and pioneering work behind the Iron Curtain amidst huge challenges, certainly had a huge impact on Barnard. Their shared isolation – given that Barnard was active at the foot of Africa, far removed from the West, which was considered to be the centre of medical progress – formed a bond between the two strangers.

The first time Barnard truly noticed Demikhov was on 10 April 1959 when Radio Moscow reported that Demikhov had again succeeded in transplanting the head of a puppy onto the body of a German Shepherd named Pirat.[12] The report indicated that the procedure had taken place 15 days earlier in Moscow and that the dog was still alive, with both heads capable of lapping up water. The second head was eventually removed 30 days after the operation.[13]

A photograph of this Demikhov experiment was also published in the media in Cape Town. The story goes that Barnard saw the photograph in the newspaper while he was in the cafeteria at Groote Schuur. He stood up and went to the animal laboratory declaring that 'anything the Russians can do, we can do too'.

That same afternoon, Barnard successfully replicated Demikhov's experiment with the help of John Terblanche and Big Vic, and Cape Town's own two-headed dog was the result. Barnard used a small dog as the donor animal and a larger dog as the base for the transplantation. The muscles and skin of the donor animal's head were attached to the larger animal's neck, just below the head. The two-headed dog survived a few days.

'Both heads drank milk from saucers,' Jannie Louw recalled later. But Louw was not happy with the experiment and asked Barnard, 'What sort of monster will you create next?'

Barnard replied, 'We'll let you know when we've done it.'

Barnard wrote in the official medical report on the operation – published in May 1960 in the *South African Medical Journal* – that the experiment indicated that the technical joining of organs, even a head, was not unattainable.

'We are investigating further the immunological reactions that follow on such transplantations. There's little doubt that tissue transplantation in various forms will become a clinical application in the foreseeable future. This will open up new fields in medicine and surgery.'

Barnard also alerted the media, which upset Louw even further. Louw put up a poster in the laboratory stating, 'Do not toy with the Delilah of the Press.'

'Chris was very angry at that and didn't speak to me for a long time,' Louw recalled later.

Animal-rights activists were also very upset, while the medical students at UCT spoofed the whole situation by creating a large, two-headed dog float made from papier-mâché for RAG.[14]

Barnard developed a desire to meet Demikhov and put his mind to facilitating this meeting. First, he applied for, and received, an Oppenheimer

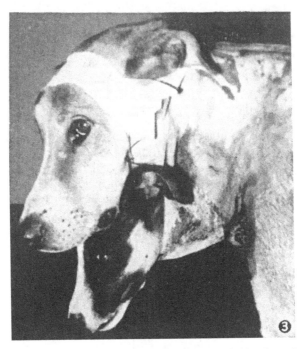

The head of a mongrel dog was transplanted onto the body of another at the
JS Marais laboratory. Within 24 hours the 'animal' reacted normally. The cerebral
and cranial functions of both heads were normal. Both heads were, for example,
observed to lap milk when this was offered.

IMAGE FROM AN ORIGINAL REPRINT COPY OF AN ARTICLE IN THE *MEDICAL PROCEEDINGS JOURNAL*, DATED 21 MAY 1960.

REPRODUCED COURTESY OF THE BEAUFORT WEST MUSEUM

bursary to enable him to travel overseas. He then began planning a trip to
Moscow, despite the significant challenges posed by such a visit behind the
Iron Curtain – it was 1960 and communism was in full force.

In addition, South Africa was severely opposed to Russia and considered Russia an arch enemy. There wasn't even a Russian Embassy in South
Africa, so Barnard had to approach the Soviet Embassy in Washington DC.

He started by writing letters to Demikhov and other high-level Russian
medical figures, explaining his research and the open-heart surgery being
done in Cape Town.

'We've performed 75 open-heart operations with a mortality rate of 8.

Those include cases of Fallot's tetralogy and others. I've heard of your work and am quite interested to experience it first hand and to meet you in person,' Barnard wrote to Demikhov.

He also explained his research and interest in cardiac surgery and transplantation, as well as his desire to learn from the Russians, to the Soviet Embassy.

'There is always room for improvement,' he wrote.

Barnard requested permission to visit several medical research centres in the Soviet Union where cardiac surgery and transplantation were being performed.

His efforts quickly drew the attention of the South African Police and he had to report for an official interview regarding the purpose of his visit. He explained to the South African authorities that it would be advantageous to South Africa if he could visit Demikhov.

Finally permission was granted from all sides and his visit to Moscow was scheduled 18–29 May 1960. Barnard would become one of very few South Africans to travel behind the Iron Curtain in those years. The visit went well. He was welcomed heartily and made at home and there was great cooperation from the Russians.

'Everything possible was done to make my visit interesting, informative and pleasant.'

Barnard attended the 27th All-Soviet Congress of Surgeons of 1960 in Moscow and made lasting friendships with some of Russia's top medical minds, including surgeons like professors Kolesnikov, Zemigov, Petrov and Demikhov himself. He continued to correspond with these professors over many years. In fact, Kolesnikov was one of the first to send Barnard a telegram congratulating him on the success of the heart transplant.

In Moscow Barnard also visited several medical research facilities, including the Sklifosovsky Institute, where he observed procedures and shared information relating to transplantation and surgical techniques.

'They showed huge interest in the work we were doing in South Africa.'

Demikhov later described himself as being a 'staunch supporter of

Barnard'.[15] Barnard wrote in 1997 that he always considered Demikhov to be an extraordinary man. He also told his family that he considered Demikhov to be his mentor.

'I always maintained that if there was a father of heart and lung transplantation, then Demikhov deserved that title,' Barnard stated.[16]

In a report to the Ernest Oppenheimer Memorial Trust following the visit, Barnard acknowledged that the Russians did have several challenges, especially in terms of antiquated equipment and technology.

'By and large, theatre technique and surgery in the USSR is of a poor quality. Their equipment is old and their techniques have been replaced long ago in the West.'[17]

Another story Barnard recounted was a general heightened tension relating to the Russians having shot down an American pilot, Gary Powers, in an American spy plane on 1 May 1960.

Inéz Barnard recalls that Christiaan visited them in Salisbury on his way back from the Soviet Union to Cape Town.

'Chris said he'd visited the Russian Bolshoi Ballet in Moscow and he was impressed by the fact that the company had used a real live horse on the stage during the ballet. He stated that this was one of the highlights of the whole trip.'

It was Demikhov who inspired Barnard and showed him that it was possible to do pioneering work outside America.

'Why should an American be the first to walk on the moon? Why can't it be a Russian? Or a South African?' Demikhov asked, according to Donald McRae's book, *Every Second Counts*.

'Okay, the first man on the moon will be a Russian, but why must the world's best surgeon be an American? Nothing is impossible,' the Russian told Barnard.[18]

The Soviets' dire lack of funding led to one humorous incident that Barnard often recounted afterwards. The Russians loved to toast their guests over drinks but, owing to funding challenges, the medical fraternity Barnard visited were making their own ethanol, which they drank instead of the usual vodka. It was cheaper and looked like vodka, but Barnard was unaware of how potent it was. The first time he drank a toast, he woke up in his hotel room in Moscow with no idea as to how he had got there.

The Americans

In America, the two top men working on heart transplantations were Norman Shumway and his friend and colleague Richard Lower. Both were affiliated to Stanford University, where they started experimenting on dogs in the 1950s.[19]

Shumway had cut his teeth in Minnesota under Wangensteen and had been in the class two years ahead of Barnard. The two were never close. Perhaps the competition between them was already building in Minnesota.

Wangensteen, who had been both Barnard's and Shumway's mentor at Minnesota, described the two as 'very good boys'. He knew that they both had huge potential, even when they were still studying under him in the 1950s.

'They both also had tons of originality.'[20]

He described Shumway as always being very analytical and investigative. 'It takes lots of determination and consecutiveness in surgical research, and Dr Shumway always had this quality in large measure.'

In later years, however, Wangensteen stated that Barnard had been the best registrar who had ever served under him.

At Stanford, Shumway made friends with Lower and the two experimented on dogs in Stanford's medical research laboratory. He later said that the best arena for training good surgeons was in the dog laboratory.[21]

While he and Lower were awaiting the outcome of one experiment, they decided to perform a heart transplant on a dog. The dog survived for eight days.[22]

In December 1959 Shumway appeared before a medical congress and reported on their dog heart transplantations.

'The transplantations showed the problem wasn't technical or physiological but immunological. The dogs behaved normally until rejection set in,' Lower stated later.

Shumway and Lower initially intended these experiments to be a technical exercise but as they continued, the dogs' survival rates and periods kept improving so the duo kept pressing on. In later years, Lower's dog patients would boast survival rates of a year or longer. He went on to establish himself in Virginia where he had one dog patient that survived for 14 months with a transplanted heart.[23]

The work done by Shumway and Lower contributed hugely to the eventual successes in human-to-human heart transplantation. For at least 10 years, this duo was at the forefront of heart transplantation, with the possible exceptions of Demikhov and three other American surgeons – Michael DeBakey and Denton Cooley in Texas and Adrian Kantrowitz in New York.

Shumway's eventual contribution to the field of organ transplantation included the transplantation of 800 human hearts.[24] By comparison, Barnard transplanted only 54 in total.

Kantrowitz also became a leading pioneer in the transplantation race, transplanting hearts into roughly 250 dogs in preparation for a human transplant, building on the published work of Shumway and Lower as well as his own research.[25] In fact, 18 months before Barnard succeeded, Kantrowitz had attempted to save a baby with a congenital birth defect by transplanting the heart of a brain-dead infant, but the baby died.

In Texas, DeBakey and Cooley were also focusing on heart surgery. Denton Cooley was a particularly hard-working surgeon, known for doing 8–12 open-heart surgeries per day. He would move between three separate theatres, doing multiple operations at the same time.

This big Texan considered the heart to be the servant of the brain – the heart was merely a pump. Cooley believed that if the brain was gone, the heart had no purpose and should be put to work elsewhere.[26]

There was no doubt, however, that Shumway and Lower were the overwhelming favourites to be the first surgeons to do a human-to-human heart transplant. If there had been any wager, the money would certainly have been on these two Stanford surgeons. No-one would have given a second thought to Barnard and the work being done in Cape Town.

However, the Americans had one huge disadvantage. American legislation defined patient death as occurring only when a heart stopped beating. Legally, brain death was not considered to be the time of death. This made organ donation incredibly difficult in America and was a huge stumbling block for the early pioneers.[27]

Raymond Hoffenberg was a senior doctor at Groote Schuur but not a member of Barnard's team. In later years, he made a name for himself in England and was knighted for his services by the Queen.

'In 1967 there were no guidelines relating to the diagnosis of the death of organ donors.'[28] Hoffenberg recalls, however, that the standard of medicine in Cape Town in the 1960s was advanced and sophisticated.

'There were well established research laboratories and an ethos that promoted research and initiative. Fulltime academic staff were often sponsored to go overseas to stay abreast of the latest medical advances. Cape Town was not an academic backwater. The environment was advantageous to innovation.'

Hoffenberg says that the Americans were worried about the ethical and legal challenges pertaining to heart transplantation and were beaten by Barnard because of this.[29]

One thing all the Americans had in common was their lack of knowledge about Christiaan Barnard. Later, when Barnard met Lower in Virginia, Lower knew very little about the South African, despite Barnard and Shumway having been at Minnesota together.

In 1964, at a conference in Port Elizabeth, Barnard predicted that the era of human heart transplantation was on the way.

'It must happen that people get new hearts. I don't know when it will happen but it must come.'[30]

His words would prove to be prophetic.

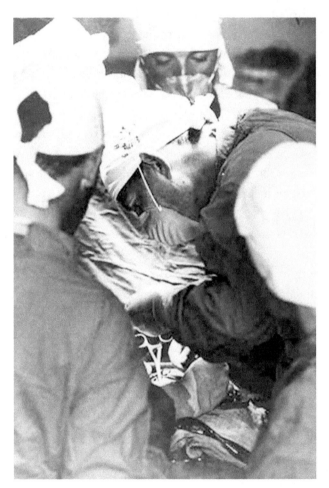

Chris Barnard has been described as one of very few surgeons who could think and work at the same time. In the first years of open-heart surgery in Cape Town, Barnard's results at Groote Schuur were astounding. Out of the first 75 open-heart surgeries, which included many severely complicated cases, only eight patients died.

CHAPTER 6

The first transplants

M EDICAL SCIENCE IS ONE GIANT PUZZLE. MANY PEOPLE WORK HARD on different sections of the puzzle and along the way larger pictures start to emerge and fall into place. However, without all the sections and the pieces, the bigger picture remains incomplete.

The same is true for organ transplantation.

Besides the pioneering work that has been described, there were many more steps taken on the way to the first successful heart transplant. These included the very first transplants, which happened to be corneas. The first cornea was transplanted successfully by an Austrian, Dr Edward Zim, in 1906. Transplanting this section of the eye creates few complications because there is no blood flow through the cornea, which means there is no rejection of the tissue.

Another important building block in the greater puzzle of organ transplantation was the study of rejection.

During the Second World War, a young Oxford zoologist, Peter Medawar, worked closely with a plastic surgeon, Thomas Gibson, experimenting with skin grafts. This was aimed at treating the burn wounds of pilots from the war.[1]

After the war, Medawar experimented further with skin grafts on animals and produced important research on rejection. He is still considered to be the father of transplantation immunology.

Unfortunately, in a book on Christiaan Barnard, one can focus on only some of these remarkable stories of medical progression.

The next piece of the puzzle was kidney transplantation.

The world's first successful kidney transplant was done in December 1954 in Boston by surgeons Joseph Murray and David Hume. The procedure took five-and-a-half hours, during which the 24-year-old patient, John Riteris, was given one of his twin brother's healthy kidneys. This meant there were no major rejection concerns. Riteris recovered and lived a long life, later marrying the nurse who had cared for him during his recovery period.

Efforts to transplant organs between people with different genetic make-up, however, are a different kettle of fish entirely and the first success in this regard was achieved only in 1959 with the help of 'heroic levels of radiation.'[2]

The field of tissue typing and matching also played a vital role in this regard. This is where the Cape Town specialist, MC Botha, played a huge role later.

In 1963 another giant in transplantation, the specialist surgeon Thomas Starzl, attempted a liver transplant. It was unsuccessful and the patient died. However, in 1967 he succeeded with this procedure.

Heart valves

The South African medical fraternity – like the rest of the country – became increasingly isolated from the rest of the world in the early 1960s following the massacre at Sharpeville.

This often meant that months of research work could be wasted when the researchers discovered that their work had already been completed and published elsewhere in the world.

South African researchers kept abreast of developments in their field as best they could through correspondence and other efforts with ex-colleagues and friends overseas.

In the late 1950s and early 1960s, the Groote Schuur cardiac research unit was becoming relatively well known across the globe for its work relating to open-heart surgery. The unit, under Barnard, developed many ground-breaking new procedures and treatments for complex heart conditions, including Fallot's tetralogy, ventricular septal defects and Ebstein's anomaly. The team also delivered excellent work with the design and application of two unique artificial heart valves.

The human heart has four valves – the pulmonic valve, the mitral valve, the aortic valve and the tricuspid valve – which are replaceable today.

There are two basic types of replacement heart valves – tissue valves and mechanical valves. Mechanical valves today are made from advanced materials like synthetic carbon and Teflon, but in the late 1950s the options were much more limited.

Barnard's Master's thesis at Minnesota was on the development of an artificial aortic valve.[3] He was on the cusp of developing the world's first artificial valve, but was beaten to it by a surgeon, Albert Starr, and an engineer, Miles Edwards, who implanted the world's first artificial heart valve, called the Starr-Edwards heart valve, into a patient in 1960.

Barnard and the Groote Schuur team pressed on, however, and in 1962 they had a breakthrough with their own unique artificial aortic valve replacement. This valve was covered with Silastic, a trade-marked mixture between silicone and plastic, which was designed to prevent blood clots, associated with pieces of metal in the body.

Louwtjie's fine needlework was a useful asset. She stitched material to the lip of the valve to provide the surgeons with a place to join the heart tissue to the valve.[4]

The Barnard team also developed an artificial mitral valve called the Barnard-Goosen valve. Goosen, who received a lot of the credit, got the idea for the valve from the exhaust system of a Morris Minor motor car. He was highly innovative and an excellent technician.

In another instance, he received his inspiration for an aortic prosthesis while he was walking to work one day.

'I came to a standstill and sketched the idea on the back of a cigarette box. Barnard had an elder brother [Johannes], an engineer at the old railway workshops in Salt River. He was known for doing good work himself with new designs for the railways. He arranged for the workshops – probably as a matter of life or death – to make my design a reality. They put in 24-hour shifts and by 4.00pm on Sunday afternoon, the first unit was completed,' Goosen recalled.[5]

For years the artificial valves designed and developed at Groote Schuur were inserted into ill patients to replace their faulty valves. One patient's new valve lasted 34 years, until he died.[6]

Deirdre Barnard

On the home front, the early 1960s were good years for the Barnard family. Ironically, it was not Christiaan Barnard who was becoming well known; instead it was his daughter, Deirdre, who became the first famous Barnard.

At the age of 12 she became a national sporting champion in water-skiing, the youngest-ever national representative.

'At least someone in the family will make it,' Chris said.[7]

Deirdre was friends with Dene Friedman – another young champion water-skier. Later Friedman – worked for Christiaan Barnard in his heart transplantation team as a technician.

Amanda Botha was the first female sports reporter appointed by the Afrikaans media group, Naspers. She got the break because, at the time, South Africa had a number of young women below the age of 18 years, who were world champions in their sport. These included Deirdre Barnard the swimmer, Karen Muirs and Ann Fairley, and the trampolin-ist Chantel Fouché. It was considered inappropriate to have older male journalists reporting on the young girls, so Botha got the job.

She met Christiaan Barnard one afternoon at DF Malan International Airport in Cape Town. Deirdre had just won a place in an international water-skiing competition.

'Chris was her coach. They spent years perfecting her skill on the lake at Zeekoevlei where the Barnards had bought a home they called The Moorings. Chris was still quite unknown while his young daughter was very famous in South Africa. At the airport, we took a photo of Chris and Deirdre and the next day he called *Die Burger* and spoke to me, requesting a copy of the photo, which I arranged. From then on, we had some contact. He told me he would call one day and then I had to drop everything and rush to Groote Schuur. He was planning something big.'

Dog heart transplantations and further research

Christiaan Barnard's interest in the concept of heart transplantation as a treatment for patients with potentially fatal cardiac disease kept increasing.[8]

In 1963, he delivered a lecture to students at the University of Pretoria in which he predicted that the 'future treatment of heart disease would include the transplantation of the human heart'.

It was in this period that Barnard's younger brother Marius arrived in Cape Town from Salisbury, where he had been a very highly regarded general practitioner. He started work at Groote Schuur on 1 July 1963.[9] He was still a general practitioner and his supervisor was Jannie Louw, who was head of the Department of Surgery.

This was a difficult time for the younger Barnard. His relationship with his elder brother was hardly perfect and it became increasingly difficult to work with Christiaan. In addition, Marius's relationship with Louw was not great either and he found himself working in the animal laboratory.

The research team had in the interim kept working hard on open-heart surgeries. Their success was so well known that the waiting time for open-heart surgery at Groote Schuur in the early 1960s was longer than two years.

Christiaan, however, was intent on pressing on with transplantation and, in 1965, he started researching the matter.[10]

Groote Schuur' s first experimental heart transplant in a dog was done in 1965 in the experimental laboratory.[11] The dog didn't survive but invaluable experience was gained.[12]

The bulk of the practical experimentation was done by Marius with the help of the laboratory assistants, Victor Pick, Hamilton Naki and John Rossouw.

'Chris was busy with lots of experiments in those days, so I undertook the majority of these experiments since I had more time available,' Marius recalls.[13]

The Barnard team continued to do experimental heart transplants on dogs for three years.

'We practised the surgical techniques in the laboratory. We were never aiming at long-term survival; all we were interested in was getting the technique perfect,' Chris said later.[14] 'As soon as it had worked out, we felt we could do heart transplants on anyone.'[15]

Between them, the Barnards and their assistants ended up doing an estimated 50 heart transplants on dogs during this period. None of the animals survived long-term.

'Many people would consider that to be a failure. We weren't successful, to be sure, but we didn't fail. We weren't looking for long-term results to study. We felt Shumway and the others had done all that already and it would have simply meant doing a lot more extra and unnecessary work. Most of our dogs could be kept alive for 18 hours, which was all we were looking for,' Marius said.[16] 'When we had done enough, we knew what had to be done.'

The theatre team's successes with open-heart surgery were world-class.

'We've just completed our 50th open-heart operation and to date we have only lost six patients,' Christiaan wrote to Wangensteen.[17]

The next step on the road to success was kidney transplants.

The first organ transplant in South Africa

When doing an organ transplant, the easiest work is in transplanting the organ. The hard work happens beforehand – the intense preparatory work needed to get a hospital ready for a procedure like a transplant. This includes building up complete surgical programmes with qualified and experienced teams, and obtaining the latest and best equipment to do the procedure. There needs to be adequate medicine and blood stocks, and specialists need a plan for post-operative treatment. With transplantation, the latter was a huge conundrum. What does one do with organ-transplant patients if the body starts to reject the tissue?

Christiaan Barnard initiated and rolled out a proactive measure to ensure the best post-operative treatment for patients at Groote Schuur – intensive-care units (ICUs). In fact, he established the practice of intensive care in South Africa. He insisted that these units be staffed with the best staff, regardless of skin colour and other non-medical issues. He also demanded that his ICU wards be desegregated, which they were.

'If a patient doesn't like it, they can go elsewhere,' he told Dene Friedmann.

'No-one ever chose to go elsewhere, because they all knew Chris was the best,' Friedmann recalls.

The other great uncertainty was donors because surgeons had no means of guaranteeing donor organs.

South Africa was 12 years behind the rest of the world when it came to organ transplantation, and the first was a kidney transplant on 25 August 1966 at the Johannesburg General Hospital, today known as the Charlotte Maxeke Johannesburg Academic Hospital.

This was performed by an academic team under the guidance of a visiting professor from the United States – the legendary transplant surgeon Tom Starzl. He was assisted by a South African professor, Bert Myburgh.[18]

The operation was performed after three years of intense preparatory work in laboratories and following the establishment of haemodialysis at the Johannesburg Academic Hospital.[19]

The story behind this remarkable bit of South African history has its origin in the United Stated in 1965. Myburgh, who was from the University of the Witwatersrand (Wits), was in the United States on a bursary and this included time at the University of Colorado in Denver, where he was a member of Starzl's faculty.[20] Starzl was known for his attempt at a liver transplantation in 1963, and many other pioneering

Who was Bert Myburgh?

Bert Myburgh was Professor of Surgery at the University of Witwatersrand. He was born in the Free State town of Linley, where he matriculated in 1944 at the age of 16. He studied at UCT to be a doctor. His academic and sporting prowess meant that he received a Rhodes Scholarship and he went to further his studies at Oxford in England. After Oxford, Myburgh returned to Wits to qualify as a surgeon. He was appointed as Professor of Surgery in 1967 and became head of Surgery in 1977. Myburgh created South Africa's first transplantation programme and did the first organ transplantation in the country in 1966. He also attempted the first liver transplantation in 1973 after a successful research programme using baboons.[23]

efforts in surgery. Myburgh, on his return to South Africa, arranged with Wits that Starzl get offered a visiting professorship.

'The duration of the Janey and Michael Miller Professorship would be one month only, during which period Myburgh wanted me to help him establish the first renal transplantation programme in Africa,' Starzl recalled in his memoir.[21]

Starzl spent the first two weeks in August 1966 training the nursing and surgical teams in Johannesburg for the operation. The training was done largely in a Johannesburg mortuary.

'Following the training, we did two kidney transplantations, with the donors coming from the families. Myburgh would continue from this foundation and make many more valuable contributions to transplantation in South Africa. He was a very talented man,' Starzl wrote.

Although the operation in Johannesburg went well, neither recipient survived very long due to rejection.[22]

Research in the United States

For the heart transplantation team in Cape Town, the technical ability to transplant a heart was no longer a problem. For years the specialists had been performing much more complicated surgeries on human hearts. The problem, however, was the team's considered inexperience with post-operative complications, mainly due to rejection.

Once again Christiaan Barnard had a solution – this time it was to be kidney transplantation. He believed that his team needed to do a kidney transplantation as a dry run for the heart transplant.

'When we were ready to do heart transplantations clinically, I decided that we needed to get experience with rejection and the management of patients who were struggling with rejection,' Barnard recalls.[24]

But first, on 3 July 1966, Marius Barnard resigned from Groote Schuur and went to the United States to study, first under Edward DeBakey and later under his Texas competitor, Denton Cooley. He was hoping to specialise in vascular surgery.[25]

Shortly after Marius left for the United States, Christiaan also decided to go to America on a three-month study trip during which he would focus on organ rejection.[26] The Americans were the world leaders in this field as a result of successes in renal transplantation.

'Kidneys had become the building blocks for heart transplantation,' Christiaan said.

He went to Virginia to study under David Hume. At least part of the reason for Christiaan's decision to study under Hume was because his star technician, Goosen, had emigrated to Virginia and based himself in Richmond.[27] Hume was one of the greatest specialists in renal transplantation and rejection, and Barnard learnt a tremendous amount from the Virginian in a very short time.

'We never slept.'[28]

One of the fundamental lessons learnt was that organ transplantation would always be followed by a struggle to combat rejection.

'Hume taught me more than anyone else how to perform successful organ transplantation. Later I would do it exactly like he did it. I also visited Tom Starzl in Colorado for two weeks,' Barnard recounts.

Starzl and Barnard had missed one another earlier in the year when Starzl had been in South Africa working with Myburgh.

During his sojourn in the United States, Barnard said nothing about heart transplantation to either Hume or Starzl. Both assumed that he was planning to establish a renal transplant unit in Cape Town.

Although Barnard's chief interest in visiting Hume in Richmond was to learn about combatting rejection,[29] this visit to Virginia would be used against him later by his greatest critics. Some claimed, and still do, that it was here that Barnard first learnt how to do heart transplants and that he 'stole' the idea from others in Virginia.

The story is complex but, in essence, unfounded. It involves Richard Lower, the great pioneer who had been doing hundreds of hours of research into heart transplantation with his friend and colleague at Stanford, Norman Shumway. By the time Barnard arrived in Virginia, Lower was already involved in a heart-transplantation programme at the university, also working under Hume. Hume was hoping that Lower would manage to bring credit to the university by being the first surgeon to do a successful human-to-human heart transplant.

Lower had developed the main technique for doing heart transplantation with Shumway. Called the Shumway-Lower technique, it had three components, a heart-lung machine, partial hypothermia, and leaving behind small sections of the patient's heart rather than removing the organ entirely.[30] Lower was still fine tuning and testing these techniques in Virginia when Barnard arrived. And it was here that he saw Lower in action, doing dog heart transplants in his laboratory in September 1966.

This happened one afternoon when Barnard was spending some time with his old colleague, Goosen, in one of the laboratories. He asked Goosen what was going on next door and Goosen replied that Lower was busy with heart transplants on dogs. Barnard wanted to know more and Goosen explained briefly.

Lower knew Barnard was a heart surgeon from South Africa, but nothing more than that. Lower agreed that Barnard could visit his laboratory and observe, which duly happened.[31]

Here things get a bit murky.

Some reports, quoting Goosen, claim that Barnard observed the procedure repeatedly in the weeks following.[32] However, Barnard later denied this.

'I watched him [Lower] for a maximum of half an hour. That was the only time I ever spent with Lower. If they say Lower taught me, I must have been a damn good student to learn it all in half an hour.'[33]

One thing was certain, though: Barnard's obsession with heart transplantation grew. He was so confident of his ability to do this, that he said as much to Goosen – that he was going to do heart transplantation on a human.

Goosen realised that Barnard was serious and warned Lower.

'How can he? He hasn't even done any research,' Lower responded, dismissing the South African out of hand.

Lower and Shumway, by this time, had already been doing research into the problem for around eight years. The Americans were completely unaware of the work being done by the research team at Groote Schuur. This was to be a big error in judgement.

At this time, Lower was probably the frontrunner in the race to do the first transplant. A few months after Barnard's visit – on 28 May 1967 – he performed a 'reverse Hardy' when he removed a human heart from a cadaver and placed it into the body of a baboon.[34]

Tissue matching and tissue typing

Christiaan Barnard had arranged for Groote Schuur to send its blood and tissue specialist, MC Botha, to Europe and America to get up to speed with the latest research regarding tissue matching.[35] This was a vital piece of the puzzle and preparation for organ transplantation. This science essentially determines whether there is a specific pattern to the rejection of foreign tissue, such as a donated organ, in an organ recipient.

Botha explained to *Die Burger* that in the 1960s there were 12 tissue factors that were reconcilable between donors and receivers of organs, but only within certain measures. It was vital to determine, as far as possible before a transplantation, if the tissues of donors and organ recipients were reconcilable or not. This reconciliation was not possible where there was a determined relationship between the factors of the recipient's tissue and that of the donated organ. One important ingredient to test tissue for compatibility is antisera, which contain antibodies that are specific to one or more antigens and can be used to pass on immunity to rejection. This valuable resource is naturally created in a pregnant woman to prevent her body from rejecting the foetus. The antisera are obtained from volunteering pregnant women through blood donations.[36]

The incompatibility of tissue was a continuing concern. Botha's three-month-long study tour to learn about the latest developments in tissue typing and matching was an effort to address this. He spent time with Jean Dausset, Paul Terasaki and Jon van Rood, three of the most influential immunologists of the time, in Amsterdam, Leiden and Los Angeles, respectively. He learnt a lot from these specialists and remained in constant contact with them for many years. This relationship proved to be invaluable to the heart-transplant team.

'Their help made it possible for us to tackle the problems that cropped up in Cape Town,' Botha said.[37]

Before a transplant, the doctors try to get tissue types to match as closely as possible to reduce the risk of rejection. Unless the genetic components are closely aligned, the body of the recipient will attack the foreign tissue and reject it. In the 1960s, and even today, the science of immunology was very tricky and fraught with many uncertainties.[38]

'The greatest problem with tissue transplantation was the scarcity of the antisera to use in the testing,' Botha said.

His network of contacts, especially Van Rood and Terasaki, enabled him to continuously exchange antisera and build up an antisera bank in the months before the transplantation.[38] This work by Botha and the network he developed was a major contributor to Groote Schuur's successes in transplantation.

While Christiaan and his team were preparing for a potential kidney transplantation, Shumway and Lower were continuing to make steady progress. On 20 September 1967, Shumway told the *Journal of the American Medical Association* that the time had come for clinical application of a human heart transplant.[39]

A few days later, on 5 October, at a congress of the American College of Surgeons in Chicago, Lower showed a film of one of his dogs that had received a heart transplant and had survived for 15 months.

Shumway repeated: 'The time has arrived to do a clinical application.'[40]

Groote Schuur's first transplantation

In South Africa, Christiaan Barnard prepared for the first kidney transplant in Cape Town. The first thing he did was to create a transplantation team.[41]

'Cape Town was still behind Johannesburg and had to still perform its first kidney transplant. Chris decided that the heart team would go over the heads of the urologists and perform the first kidney transplant in Cape Town. There was strong opposition to that, especially from the Department of Urology, but Chris went ahead regardless,' Marius recalls.

After his three months under Cooley and a visit from Inéz, Marius decided to return home.

'Jannie Louw refused to offer me a job and I would have returned to South Africa unemployed. Chris recognised my financial position and offered me a position as a consultant in the transplantation team.'

By this stage, Barnard's team had grown. Now there were four surgeons working under Christiaan Barnard, including Marius. The chief of the lot was the brilliant Rodney Hewitson.

Joseph 'Ozzy' Ozinsky

The Jewish Ozinsky was born in 1927 and arrived in South Africa six months later after his family fled persecution in Europe. He completed his schooling at SACS in Cape Town, where he was a Queen Victoria scholar – a high academic honour. He received training in the United Kingdom and further training in Durban. He returned to Cape Town, initially to the Red Cross Children's Hospital and later Groote Schuur. On Barnard's return to Groote Schuur, Ozzy became the chief cardiac anaesthetist. From 1967, he and Barnard's team performed about 1 000 open-heart surgeries. Ozinsky retired in 1992.

He hoarded everything, from medical records to adverts and anything that he thought may have a use later. But it never did prove useful.

Ozinsky died in August 2017, months before the 50th anniversary of the first heart transplant. He was 90 years old.[42]

'Rodney was an immense help to us all and was a great surgeon to work with. The second surgeon in the department was Terry O'Donovan. I was the inexperienced third,' Marius writes in his book.

The team was supported by three registrars, Bertie 'Bossie' Bosman, Francois Hitchcock and Coert Venter; the last named was from Pretoria and known to be quite a maverick with a surgical blade.

Two other departments that were critical cogs in the transplantation machine were the Department of Cardiology under Velva 'Val' Schrire and the Department of Anaesthesiology. The senior anaesthestist was Joseph 'Ozzy' Ozinsky. He never paid much attention to Barnard's angry outbursts during operations and would often pretend that he didn't understand the professor at all.

Sister Amelia Rautenbach's nickname was Pittie because her dad had always called her 'Mieliepit', the Afrikaans word for a corn kernel. Pittie

Velva 'Val' Schrire

Velva Schrire, another extraordinary medical practitioner and head of the Cardiology Clinic at Groote Schuur, is considered to be the father of cardiology in South Africa.

Schrire matriculated in 1933 from Kimberley Boys' High School with five distinctions. He went on to become the Dux scholar at UCT where he won 10 gold medals and four scholarships. In 1949, he was awarded the prestigious Nuffield Travelling Fellowship in London. While in London, he became a Member of the Royal College of Physicians, another great honour.

Schrire returned to South Africa, where he established the Cardiology Unit at Groote Schuur. He became world famous in medical circles in his own right and was a brilliant surgeon, but reticent and not fond of the media or public attention. He is described as a Renaissance man who had a broad knowledge of all things and who was blessed with a photographic memory.

Schrire was known to have seen more than 20 000 patients per year at Groote Schuur and he could recall each patient's name and medical details.[43] His patients loved him and found him to be friendly and sympathetic, while his critics considered him taciturn and unapproachable. This did not faze Velva for whom the patients always came first. He was the specialist who recommended Louis Washkansky for a heart transplant.[44]

was also from the Karoo and would eventually work side by side with Barnard for more than 20 years.[45]

'Perhaps we got along because we were both from the Karoo and people from the Karoo are tough.'

At 5.00am on 8 October 1968, a Sunday, Pittie was awakened by the telephone.[46] It was the hospital. Prof Barnard was going to do a kidney transplant at 6.00am.

The team of specialists had been preparing for a while and had held weekly meetings at which each one's role and responsibility was determined.

Christiaan Barnard recounts his one and only kidney transplant: 'Only by October 1967, a year after my return to South Africa, were we ready to do a kidney transplant. And so Edith Black became our first patient at Groote Schuur.'[47]

Mrs Black, a 36-year-old housewife from Plumstead, Cape Town, would become the first person in Cape Town to get a kidney transplant.[48]

The Barnard team's kidney transplant was a huge success and three weeks after the operation, Mrs Black left the hospital and continued her life.[49] She lived for another 20 years.[50]

The valuable experience with the kidney transplant gave the Barnard team further insight into the realities of organ transplantation. Some of the most valuable lessons involved getting permission from donors' families and dealing with the risk of infection and post-operative treatment.

For years the heart team from Groote Schuur boasted about their proud kidney-transplantation record and would claim that they had the best survival rate in kidney transplantation in the world, a 100% success rate. The team did, however, only ever do one kidney transplant!

The team's success with this first transplant gave them the courage and confidence to go ahead with heart transplantation. Christiaan Barnard recalled that with this operation 'all the machinery of the transplantation team worked perfectly ... we were ready to do a heart transplant'.[51]

Kidney transplantation research was also ongoing at another Cape Town hospital, Karl Bremer, where hundreds of experimental kidney transplants had been done on baboons. These experiments were being done under the auspices of Stellenbosch University in collaboration with the Brady Institute of Urology from Johns Hopkins Hospital in the United States.[52] It was to Karl Bremer that Denise Darvall's kidney would be sent for transplantation into a young boy named Jonathan van Wyk, who had been waiting for a transplant for three months.

Karl Bremer's researchers believed that baboons were more suitable for experimental work than dogs because of their blood compatibility with humans. Regardless, farmers were happy about this decision and were trapping and selling baboons to Karl Bremer at R10 a head.

After the kidney transplant, there was no stopping Christiaan Barnard. 'The only thing he could talk about was the heart transplant,' says Marius.[53]

Shumway and Barnard

On 21 November 1967, Shumway again wrote in the *Journal of the American Medical Association* that the way was open for human heart transplantation. He went on to say that his experience, achieved through animal heart transplantations, gave him the confidence that his team would be able to care for a patient with a transplanted heart.[54] He said that Stanford would do a heart transplant as soon as a patient and donor became available.

South African doctors at the time were approached for comment and their comment was that Shumway's promise was all good and well, but that the three main challenges remained: storing the heart once it was removed from the donor body, resuscitating the heart once it was transplanted and, finally, rejection.[55]

One surgeon from Cape Town, whose comments would be reported anonymously, remarked cuttingly: 'They are no further than we are. Across the world there are doctors working with the same issues. We ourselves have been experimenting on animals for three or four years.'

This anonymous doctor was Christiaan Barnard.[56]

By December 1967, between them, the Barnard brothers had transplanted an estimated 48 dog hearts in the research laboratory. The exact figures are unknown because, as Marius Barnard explained later, they never kept a record of the numbers.

Marius did 90% of the operations.[57]

Chris Barnard wrote in *One Life* that they had done 48 dog heart transplantations.

'In 90% of the experiments the hearts started beating regularly. We used a technique based on the one developed by Shumway and Lower, who had been testing it on hundreds of dogs. If we added their findings to our own, it made little sense to continue doing more experiments. Scientific research is based on the principle that one uses existing knowledge to acquire additional knowledge.'

Either way, the Barnards did considerably fewer experiments, easily 250 fewer than Shumway and Lower, and hundreds less than Kantrowitz, who was also still hard at work.

The Americans were also able to keep their animal patients alive for a year or longer following their transplants. The Barnards' best survival period was 10 days.[58]

Schrire pointed this out to Barnard who replied: 'We aren't trying to make the dogs live longer. I can't nurse a dog like a person. We can't treat dogs with immune-suppressant drugs like we can humans. We know how to treat human patients.'

In November 1967, Christiaan Barnard officially announced that he was ready to perform a human-to-human heart transplant.[59] This statement went largely unnoticed, even by his medical colleagues.[60] His mark was drawn in the sand, however, and his homework had been done.

'By then we had already been working on heart transplants in the laboratory for years and we had experience with kidney transplantation. We were well prepared.'[61]

The legal problem

The race was on to do the first successful heart transplant. The work had been done and the teams were ready but there were two uncertainties that remained unknown and unpredictable: the donor and the legal aspect, that is, when can a donor be classified dead?

Heart surgeons have to transplant a donor heart as quickly as possible because once a donor has died, there is very little time before the heart becomes irrevocably damaged.

But when is a donor dead? In America and Europe, it was generally accepted that patients were dead when their hearts stopped beating. This, however, posed a problem because the heart starts dying as soon as it stops beating, making a transplant impossible.

The alternative was to accept that brain-dead patients were dead. In this case, the organs of these patients could be kept alive artificially until the surgeons were ready to harvest them for transplantation.

Uncertainty around this debate was a grave concern because if surgeons removed the heart from a patient who was considered to be still alive, those surgeons would be committing murder.

Americans, in particular, were greatly concerned about the legalities and were, accordingly, wary about performing heart transplants. In America, brain death was not considered to be clinical death, and surgeons were aware that if they acted incorrectly, it could mean the end of their careers, if not jail time.

In South Africa, medical legislation was slightly less draconian and more open-minded. This gave the Groote Schuur team an added boost. Barnard had, nevertheless, consulted a professor in forensic pathology, Lionel Smith, and asked for clarity on this issue.[62]

Smith explained that in South Africa the authorities had purposely left the definition of clinical death vague. This meant that it was up to the doctor to decide if a patient was clinically dead, and brain-death declarations were legal.

A controversy that faced the Barnard team, which their American counterparts didn't have to worry about, was the impact of apartheid. Schrire was concerned that if the donor and/or patient were not white, the fallout from a race issue could be enormous. Schrire and Barnard were worried that the world could accuse Groote Schuur of experimenting on black patients in this situation, so they reached an agreement that both the donor and the patient had to be white.

Had they not taken this decision, they may well have done the world's first heart transplantation two weeks earlier, when a donor heart from a non-white donor became available.[63]

By the end of 1967, when they were ready for the first heart transplant,

Barnard and his team had performed more than 1 000 open-heart operations. The waiting list was still far in excess of 2 000 patients and the team could perform only four per day.[64]

A Cape Town grocer, Louis Washkansky, was taken to Groote Schuur Hospital on 14 September 1967. Here he was treated by Schrire, who realised there was not much more they could do for him – he was dying. On 10 November 1967, Schrire referred Washkansky to Barnard for a heart transplant.

PART TWO

The operation,
3 December 1967

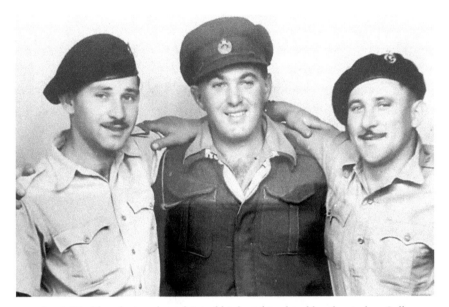

Louis Washkansky (on the right) and his best friend and brother-in-law, Solly Sklar (centre) and another friend, Morris Levin, in their army uniforms, in Italy, 1943. Washkansky was 'a delightful man' recalls Georgie de Klerk, the nursing sister who tended to him at Groote Schuur.

CHAPTER 7

The characters

Louis Washkansky was born in Lithuania in 1914. When he was nine years old, he, together with his mother, brothers and sisters, emigrated to Cape Town to join their father. Old man Washkansky had gone to Cape Town ahead of his family and started up a grocery store in Gardens near the city centre.[1]

The Jewish family made their new home in Sea Point and quickly became part of the growing Jewish community at the foot of Signal Hill.

Louis, a big bear of a man, was called Washy by his friends. He was an enthusiastic weightlifter and wrestler and spent his free time coaching kids at the local Maccabi wrestling club. It was here that Washy met his best friend Solly Sklar.[2] Solly had followed a similar route to Washy – his family had also fled from persecution in Lithuania and had settled in Cape Town. The two become firm friends.

Washy could always look after himself, no matter what obstacles came his way.

'Put him in the middle of the desert without water and Louis would come riding out on a camel loaded up with beer,' according to Solly.

The two men joined the South African Armed Forces in 1940 as members of the Engineering Corps and went to North Africa to fight the Germans and the Italians. They shared a trench for five years of war and Solly recalls that his old friend was courageous but with a soft heart for the underdog.[3]

'Louis was clever and handy. He once made a contraption with which he could make his own brew, with kick, from orange peels and raisins.

It had pipes and tubes like a real chemistry set. After five days, the brew would bubble up and a green liquid would drip into a can. Louis swopped this contraption for some eggs that he shared with us all. Then he came upon a depot where the Germans had left behind some flour. This he exchanged for an ox. He knew the Military Police would find out about the animal so he wiped out all tracks after he'd transported the animal with a truck. He said that if someone asked where the animal came from, we had to say it had shown up at morning roll call. The entire company had fresh meat for a change instead of the usual canned beef. Everyone loved the guy.'[4]

Washy convinced the army that he needed soft leather boots for his problematic feet which had kept him from the infantry and seen him join the Engineering Corps instead.

He made a deal with the army. He would pay for his own leather boots and the army would repay him after the war at a rate of nine pence per day for the duration of his military service.

Washy ended up with a pair of black knee-high Italian leather boots that he picked up in Abyssinia. He would walk around with a medical certificate that stated other boots were bad for his feet.

'Nobody could get him out of them, not even the MPs. If there was a parade, there Washy would be with his knee-high boots. He wore them the entire war and with our demobilisation he put in his claim for boot leather and the army paid him out a lump sum in full. The money he used to throw a party for the entire company,' Solly recalls.[5]

This party was held in the old Zionist hall in Hope Street.[6]

In 1947, Washkansky opened his own grocery store and married Solly's sister, Anne Sklar.[7]

However, his hard-living, unhealthy lifestyle of drinking and smoking finally caught up with him and he had his first heart attack in December 1960. He also developed diabetes. For seven years he struggled with the disease in his chest and increasingly difficult breathing.

In January 1967, his doctor referred him to the cardiology clinic at Groote Schuur. By late autumn, Washkansky's condition had deteriorated and he was hovering at death's door. This was when Schrire had him admitted. Anne Washkansky said that the scale was balanced against Louis from the start.

It quickly became clear that without a heart transplant he wouldn't be alive much longer. But such a procedure had never been performed before.

'It was Louis' phenomenal courage and will to live that motivated the doctors to go ahead with the procedure,' Anne said.

'The man's will to live is fantastic,' Christiaan told Anne.

'My husband showed such a fighting spirit that the medical experts approached him and told him about transplantation and what it would entail. He grabbed the opportunity immediately and didn't even need the two days Prof Barnard offered him to think about it. By this time his life was hanging by a thread. He'd been dying for two months already and knew the operation was his only chance at a longer life,' Anne said.

Anne continued: 'Barnard guaranteed him a new life if the operation was a success. We had no idea when the operation would take place. I was scared but my husband's faith in the medical personnel inspired me too. He kept saying, "I'll beat the odds, I'll pull through."'

Later the medical team discovered that Washkansky's heart had only about 10% of function left, with large parts of the heart muscle damaged beyond repair.[8]

Following Schrire's recommendation, Barnard agreed Washkansky was a good candidate to undergo the procedure.[9]

The Groote Schuur transplant team was ready to proceed. On 22 November, Washkansky nearly got his new heart but problems with the donor heart sank this opportunity.

'It was cancelled at the last minute. It was an unforeseen thing and was the only time I saw my husband's spirit sink,' Anne recalled.

On Saturday afternoon, 2 December 1967, Anne visited her husband in hospital as usual. In the weeks that he'd been lying in the hospital, she had smuggled him homemade food and tried endlessly to keep him positive. Solly often helped his sister. But Washy was nearing the end and there was still no certainty about when a donor heart might become available.

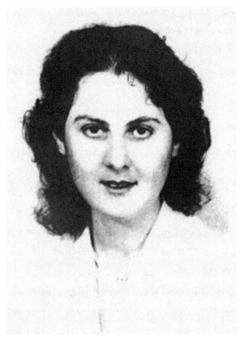

25-year-old Denise Darvall became a central figure in the world's first
heart transplant in 1967 after she and her mother, Myrtle, were struck down
fatally by a car as they were crossing Main Road, Observatory, Cape Town.

PHOTOGRAPH COURTESY OF THE HEART OF CAPE TOWN MUSEUM

'He was angry that Saturday afternoon and said all the doctors had entered his room and greeted him as they left for the weekend. He was convinced they'd all gone fishing and he thought there was no chance that the operation would take place that weekend.'

Denise Darvall

The Darvall family lived up a side street near Jan van Riebeek High School in Tamboerskloof. They had been living in a two-bedroomed flat in Mirano Court for a while.

Saturday, 2 December 1967, was a glorious day in Cape Town. Like most Capetonians, the Darvalls enjoyed leaving the confines of the apartment in fine weather, and this particular Saturday, they decided to visit friends in Milnerton, a suburb roughly 12 kilometres from the city centre on the way to Blouberg.

The 25-year-old Denise Ann Darvall was a banking clerk and the family's main breadwinner. She was a great fan of Barbara Cartland novels and didn't much appreciate the latest music fads such as Elvis or the Beatles. Instead, she rather enjoyed Joan Sutherland and opera music.

The Darvalls were not well off, but for Denise – the family called her Denny – things were looking up. She had just been promoted at the bank and was getting paid R120 per month. After the raise, she bought herself a new blue and white Ford Anglia, which became the family of five's prized possession.[10]

That morning, Denise, her 53-year-old mom Myrtle, 66-year-old dad Edward and youngest brother, Keith, who was 14 years old, left in the Anglia with Denny behind the wheel and her mom seated next to her. Denny's other brother, 17-year-old Stephen, chose to stay at home.

He would never again see his sister or mother alive.

The four Darvalls left their apartment in Gilmourhill Road at 2.45pm. They never liked to arrive at friends empty handed, so they decided to stop for a cake at Wrench's Bakery in Main Road, Observatory. Joseph Copenberg's bakery had an excellent reputation for freshly baked goods and the family decided to buy one of the bakery's famous caramel cakes for 80 cents.

Denise drove to the bakery, a detour of around 3.2 kilometres. She drove southwards down Main Road, with Table Mountain on the right, and parked on the side of the road opposite the bakery. There was a concrete island in the centre of the road separating the opposite lanes.

Denny and her mother got out of the car and went to the bakery. The men remained in the car.[11]

Myrtle and Denise were on their way back and were crossing the road when an approaching truck blocked the view of the oncoming traffic in the second lane behind the truck. The truck driver was trying to beat the traffic light and had accelerated when the lights changed from orange to red.

The accident

Frederick Prins (36 years old) had been married for two years. He'd had a few drinks and was on his way to his home in Rosebank. He was meant to pick up his wife from her job at Groote Schuur Hospital, but decided he had to return to work first to ensure that a scheduled delivery had gone out on time. He turned his car around and drove back to his place of work.[12] He was in a hurry when he overtook the truck on Main Road.

Denny and Myrtle never even saw the motor vehicle coming. Just after 3.30pm, Prins hit the two Darvalls. Denise's dad and youngest brother heard the accident happen – an enormous bang.

The family's matriarch died on impact. Denise was thrown high into the air and coming down her head struck the wheel of a parked vehicle. She cracked open her skull and sustained serious injuries.[13] However, her heart kept beating as she lay in the road with severe head injuries.

In a strange coincidence, Anne Washkansky drove past the accident scene on her way home from visiting her husband in hospital. Groote Schuur is about a kilometre further down the road.

Edward Darvall fought his way through the crowd to get to his family's side. Dazed, he got into the ambulance that arrived and went with Denise to Groote Schuur. Johan Naudé was the doctor on duty when Denise arrived at Groote Schuur's casualty ward.

'I was on duty when a young woman with a fatal head injury was admitted. I connected her to a ventilator and cared for her as best I could. We all knew the cardiac team was on call to do a transplantation and so I called the cardiologists and the neurosurgeons.'

Coert Venter was the cardiologist on duty at Groote Schuur that afternoon and it was he who informed Christiaan Barnard that a potential donor was at the hospital.

Prins called his wife from Woodstock Police Station at 3.30pm and was released on bail of R50.[14]

CHAPTER 8

The heart transplant

A
T APPROXIMATELY 8.00PM ON SATURDAY EVENING, CHRISTIAAN
Barnard's phone rang for the first time at his home in Zeekoevlei,
about 15 kilometres from Groote Schuur Hospital.

'Chris Barnard.'

'Prof, I think we have a donor.' It was Coert Venter.

'Who is it?'

'A young girl who was hit by a car. She has serious brain damage.'

'What are the neurosurgeons saying?'

'Dr Rose-Innes is looking at her now.'

'Tell him to call me as soon as possible.'

Barnard waited a while until the suspense became too much and he
called the hospital for a progress update, but Venter was unavailable. Ten
minutes later Venter called back. Chris could hear in his voice that they
had something.

'I have the donor in our ward,' said Venter.

'Already? In C-2?'

'Yes.'

'What's her blood type?'

'It's okay, it's O.'

'Did you get permission?'

'No, I haven't got permission yet.'

Barnard paused a moment, angry: 'How can you take in a patient
without first getting permission?'

'I'll find out about the permission.'

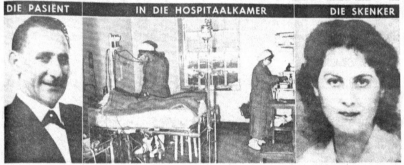
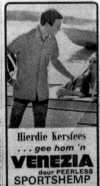

Newspapers in Cape Town broke the story of the world's first heart transplant on Monday 4 December 1967. The boy pictured at the bottom of the page is Jonathan van Wyk, who received Denise Darvall's kidney in an operation at Karl Bremer hospital.

REPRODUCED COURTESY OF *DIE BURGER*.

'I'm coming immediately,' Barnard replied.

Christiaan said goodbye to Louwtjie, jumped into his red Alfa and sped off to Groote Schuur.[1] The memory of the close call weeks earlier spurred him on.

Edward Darvall was still waiting for news of his daughter. He already knew that his wife was dead.

'I was sitting there when Dr Bosman and Dr Venter came to see me and said they wanted to speak to me. They said they wanted to be honest, they had done everything they could for Denise, but there was nothing left to do. There was no hope for her.'

Bosman spoke with Darvall about organ donation and wanted to know if Denise's heart and kidneys could be used to save the lives of two other patients who were desperately ill.

Edward needed only a few minutes to make his decision. He was reminded of a moment when his daughter had used some of her first pay cheque to buy him a new nightgown. He recalled how his Denny always gave freely to others.

'They asked me to allow them to transplant my daughter's heart into another patient. I said if there was nothing more to be done for her, they had to try to save the man's life.'

At Groote Schuur, Christiaan Barnard went straight to Ward C-2, bounding up the short flight of stairs. He found Venter and Bosman beside the bed where Denise Darvall was lying, connected to machines in one of the 11 rooms in the ward. The two registrars told their boss that the neurosurgeons had confirmed that there was nothing more that could be done for Denise Darvall.

'Well, they didn't tell me,' Barnard said. 'Get Rose-Innes and Schrire back here and tell them we need a final look. Did we get permission?' he asked.

'Yes, also for the kidneys,' Bosman replied.

Rose-Innes and Schrire were called to Ward C-2. It was important for Barnard to get Rose-Innes's permission in person, while Schrire needed to confirm that there was no cardiological damage to the donor's heart.

Barnard then gave the green light to call in the entire transplantation team. 'Call them in. All of them.'

Bossie left to make the calls, more than 30 of them all across the Peninsula.

The cardiology unit had a list of the names of all members of the heart-transplantation team in the on-call room. For the previous three weeks, there had been a standing arrangement that everyone on this list had to let the sister on duty know about their movements when they were not on duty and they had to be contactable at all times.

Calls went out to private homes and private parties – like the one the three theatre sisters were attending dressed in vintage bathing suits. The police had to radio Rodney Hewitson, second in charge after Barnard, because he was camping and was unreachable by phone.

Dr MC Botha, the pathologist in charge of the Cape Provincial Blood Laboratory, was called at his home in Rosebank.[2] He had already been working for weeks in the laboratory on samples of Washkansky's tissue, so he wasn't caught off guard when he got his call. This tissue typing was done in conjunction with the Western Cape Blood Transfusion Services.

'We arranged that there would be 10 bottles of the correct type of blood on hand every day,' Botha said.

The team at Groote Schuur needed to know if he could, as a matter of urgency, do the necessary tissue typing on Darvall's tissue samples. He indicated that he needed at least two hours and immediately left for his laboratory, where two assistants were standing by with a blood sample taken from Denise Darvall. He confirmed that the tissue match would not be a problem: Darvall's blood group was type O, while Washkansky's was A, and these blood groups are compatible.

Botha then called Karl Bremer Hospital in Bellville, where there was a desperately ill coloured boy named Jonathan van Wyk, who was waiting for a kidney donor. He determined that Darvall's kidneys were also a match for Van Wyk, so Dr Johan 'Guy' de Klerk was dispatched to Groote Schuur to retrieve the kidneys for their young patient.[3]

Doctors Rose-Innes and Schrire had arrived in Ward C-2. The

neurosurgeon Rose-Innes confirmed that Darvall was brain dead and said, 'You may go ahead.' Schrire confirmed that the donor heart was healthy but said, 'It's fine for now, but damage is to be expected the longer you wait.'

'Okay, we're not waiting any longer,' Barnard said.

He walked out and carried on down the ward to Washkansky's room where the nurses were shaving his chest in preparation for the procedure.

'Is this it, Doc?' asked Washkansky.

Barnard nodded and asked, 'How do you feel?'

'Like a boxer entering a ring without knowing who the opponent will be.'

Barnard said nothing.

Washkansky went on, 'How're my odds looking, Doc? They're always changing at the last minute. Are they changing in my favour or against?'

'In your favour,' Barnard said.

The sisters started shaving his stomach. Barnard could see no sign of fear in Washkansky's eyes.

'Please tell Anne not to worry. It's in the bag.'

'Good,' said Barnard and went to call Anne to inform her that the operation was going ahead.

'He said to tell you not to worry.'

'If it helps, tell him I'm not worried,' replied Anne. She had decided to stay at home.

Then Barnard went to the theatre changing rooms as the heart transplant team continued to arrive.

In the changing rooms, his brother Marius and doctors Bosman, Terry O'Donovan and Hitchcock were all getting dressed for theatre in their white pants, surgical vests and boots prior to scrubbing up. They discussed the coming procedure.

Marius and O'Donovan were going to be in charge of the donor in Theatre B. Marius told his elder brother that he and Terry would get Darvall ready but that Chris should remove the donor heart personally to get the feel for the organ before transplanting it.

The discussion ended and Christiaan continued to the senior surgeon's changing room, which he shared with Hewitson. Here the surgeon from the Karoo spent some time by himself contemplating what was to come, while Hewitson was still en route. Christiaan found himself on the white bench in the changing room when self-doubt started to rise. He had to fight the thoughts of doubt and worry creeping in.

'Professor Barnard, may we walk through here?'

It was Sister Tollie Lambrechts. She and Dene Friedmann were moving Barnard's original heart-lung machine from the locked storeroom where it was kept to Theatre A, where it was to be set up for Washkansky. When Chris saw that machine, the machine with which he'd had such success, all self-doubt vanished.

'Go ahead, Sister.'

At 11.45pm Denise Darvall was in Theatre B, still dependent on artificial respiration.

Sisters Rossouw and Rautenbach were assisting in Theatre B.[4]

'I felt so sad, I struggled to look at that lovely girl and had to swallow to prevent myself from crying, but there was too much to do,' Rautenbach recalled.[5]

'Prof Barnard walked in and asked if everything was ready. He was a brilliant captain, in charge of every last detail.'[6]

Ten minutes later, Washkansky was pushed into Theatre A where sisters Peggy Jordaan, Tollie Lambrechts and Joan Fox Smith were on duty. Barnard returned to Theatre A where Ozzy Ozinsky was preparing to anaesthetise Washkansky.

Before going under, Washy wanted to know if Barnard had told Anne everything would be okay. Barnard nodded.

Barnard went back to Theatre B where the assistant anaesthesiologist, Cecil Moss (a former Springbok rugby player) was checking Denise's electrocardiogram (ECG) readings and feeding tubes. Marius and O'Donovan were preparing the chest for surgery. It was a tricky situation. Darvall was brain dead but Barnard was not comfortable opening her yet and wanted to wait until her heart stopped beating before removing it. But the process had to be timed precisely because they also needed to wait until Washkansky was ready to receive his new heart.

Two interlinked rooms separated Theatre A from Theatre B. One was the instrument room, the other, the scrub room. Here Barnard found Rodney Hewitson who had just arrived from Hermanus. The two of them went on to Theatre A where Washkansky was lying. Hewitson joined Hitchcock at the table and the two surgeons started with the procedure to put Washkansky on bypass.

Barnard went back to Theatre B and Denise. Marius told him that Darvall's condition was deteriorating rapidly. O'Donovan and Coert Venter concurred. Marius wanted to take Denise off the machines and put her on bypass, but Chris insisted that they wait until Washkansky was ready for bypass himself. He hurried back to Theatre A – a trip he would make many times that night.

Back in Theatre A, Hewitson opened up Washkansky's chest. The grocer's sick heart was visible for the first time. The badly damaged heart had Hewitson looking at Barnard for a moment.

'You ever seen anything like that?'

'Never,' said Hewitson.

Later Chris said that when he saw Washkansky's heart, he knew that no treatment other than a transplant could have helped him.[7]

Chris instructed the team in Theatre A to get Washkansky ready for the heart-lung machine and returned to Theatre B, where Marius, who had had his back to Theatre A, turned as his brother entered and asked, 'Now?'

'Now,' Chris replied.

The machine keeping Denise alive was switched off, but her heart kept on beating. It was refusing to give up. She had already been declared brain dead and, surgically, the right thing to do was to remove the heart while it was still beating and at its strongest. But the team waited. O'Donovan said that he wasn't cutting until the ECG was flat. Christiaan nodded in agreement.

'We must wait until it stops,' he said.

'There was, at the time, a moral obligation on us to remove the donor heart only once it was "dead" and this was the way we would proceed for the first few transplants,' O'Donovan recalled later.[8]

Denise's blood pressure gradually fell as her heart kept beating stubbornly for another 15 minutes, until the ECG line went flat. Then her heart stopped. It was 2.32am.

'Let's wait till we're sure it won't beat again,' said Barnard.[9]

At this stage, the ECG was showing no heart activity. The team waited another five minutes before Christiaan finally said to O'Donovan, 'Start cutting, Terry.'

The official record of the operation describes this as follows: 'The donor was declared dead after the electrocardiogram showed no activity for five minutes and after a lack of any spontaneous respiratory movement.'[10]

Barnard hurried back to Theatre A.

'Are you ready to go on bypass, Rodney?' he asked, before rushing back to the scrub room to start scrubbing up for surgery. Until now, Barnard had been running up and down and hadn't touched one of the two patients. Now he had to get actively involved. While washing up he heard O'Donovan and his brother starting to saw through Darvall's chest.

Back in Theatre B, Cecil Moss was monitoring the donor heart. He worked closely with Ozinsky who was based in Theatre A.

Next was the danger period and the second great challenge. Denise's heart had to be kept alive until it was time to transplant it into Washkansky's chest. An organ intended for transplantation degenerates rapidly if it is left inside the body of a deceased person. The cells begin dying due to a lack of oxygenated blood and this damage is irreparable.

The surgeons had to work fast to get the donor heart on bypass. Heparin was injected to prevent the blood from clotting. Since her heart had stopped beating, catheters had to be inserted, and oxygenated blood and other nutrients had to be infused into the heart to prevent it from dying. When everything was ready, Marius instructed the technicians in Theatre B – Alistair Hope and Nic Vermaak – to switch on the heart-lung machine and place Darvall and her heart onto bypass.

Barnard finished scrubbing up and put on the green gown and thin rubber gloves that surgeons wore for theatre. He made one last visit to Theatre A.

'Everything ready, Rodney?

Hewitson nodded.

'Johan?'

'Ja, Professor,' nodded Van Heerden, the chief technician.

'Switch on.'

Washkansky went onto bypass, his ruined heart fighting gamely, perfused with oxygenated blood from the machine. Van Heerden's assistant, Dene Friedmann, constantly called out the blood-pressure readings for the surgeons from the heart-lung machine.

'Everything okay, Johan?'

'Ja, Professor.'

'Ozzy?'

'Everything okay. But perhaps you better go fetch that other heart before someone else claims it,' the anaesthesiologist noted drily.

In Theatre B, the donor heart had been freed from its moorings by O'Donovan by the time Chris arrived back.

'There you go,' said O'Donovan.

The heart-lung machine was switched off. Chris excised the heart himself, cutting the eight vessels entering the heart with a small pair of scissors that Sister Rautenbach handed him. Chris then placed his hands into the chest cavity and gently lifted out the small organ and placed it in a dish containing a salt solution.

'Marius held a small dish that was filled with the ice-cold solution of Ringer's lactate. I lifted the heart with both hands and placed it in the dish. The blood in the heart turned the salty solution pink. I couldn't see the heart, just the catheters that hung over the sides of the dish. Here we go, I said, taking the dish, and began walking the 31 steps from the one operating table to the other,' Chris recalled in later years.

Sister Rautenbach remembered the feeling when Denise Darvall's body was taken away with its empty chest.[11] 'We were all silent.'

All the Theatre B staff trooped over to Theatre A when their tasks were done and sat in the packed gallery with the other spectators to watch the rest of the transplantation.

The donor heart arrived in Theatre A at 3.01am in a silver dish and was handed to Sister Peggy Jordaan, the chief scrub sister who was waiting at the foot of the operating table. Chris connected the donor heart to a line from the heart-lung machine in Theatre A to perfuse it with oxygenated blood and prevent as much damage as possible before it could be joined to the remnants of Washkansky's heart.

Next, Washkansky's diseased heart had to be removed. This was the moment of reckoning. A first operation like this one is always especially difficult because surgeons don't know exactly what to expect, but Barnard had enough confidence to take the leap into the great unknown. Few surgeons would take unnecessary chances with a patient's life but, in Barnard's opinion, it was critical to take a chance if Washkansky were to survive.

But the reality was that – even though he had a sick heart – Washkansky was still alive. Once his heart was cut out, however, there would be no going back. If the operation didn't work, Washkansky would be dead.

Barnard started cutting. Washkansky's sick old heart was excised from the chest cavity but Barnard left behind the roof of the atria. This would act as a foundation onto which the new heart would be joined. This was a technique that Shumway and Lower's research indicated would be most effective.

Finally, Christiaan placed his hands into Washkansky's chest and lifted out the old diseased heart. He placed it in a dish that Sister Lambrechts was holding.

'The cavity left behind was enormous. This was something few people had ever seen, a person without a heart, being kept alive by a machine only eight steps away.'

The point of no return had been reached.

Bosman took the dish containing the donor's heart and placed it on Washkansky's leg.

'I took Denise Darvall's small, pink heart – firm and cold – in my hands. The next great challenge was to join the donor heart to Washkansky's venous system. The donor heart was prepared for joining with Washkansky's body. I stared at it a moment and wondered if it would ever work. It looked so small, too small to ever be able to tackle the challenges that would be thrown at it. The heart of a woman is 20% smaller than that of a man and, in addition, Washkansky's heart had left behind a hollow that was twice as large as the normal chest cavity,' Barnard recalled.

He placed the donor heart into the large cavity. It appeared lost and ineffectual. Barnard and Hewitson started joining the heart chambers, the aorta and pulmonary arteries to Washkansky's body[12] in a process called anastomosis[13]. This was the most painstaking and time-consuming part of the transplantation.

Once the anastomosis had been completed, bleeding checks done and all air expelled, the aorta was unclamped and the heart became one with Washkansky's body for the first time. It was 5.15am.

Barnard gave the order to the team to start rewarming Washkansky's body. It had ben cooled as part of the bypass process. At 5.43am the transplantation was complete.

All the theatre sisters and the other surgeons from Theatre B were seated in the gallery, waiting, some with balled fists, filled with tension at the proceedings in front of them. Washkansky's personal doctor had also spent the five hours of the operation perched on a high chair.

It was the moment of truth. Would a heart that had been allowed to die, start up again? The spectators in the gallery leaned forward.

Barnard called for the paddles of the defibrillator. The entire room was quiet. The moment had arrived – would Denise Darvall's heart beat again? It had not beaten since it had been removed from her chest hours earlier.

Electrodes were connected to the heart through which an electrical current of 20 watts per second was sent into Washkansky's new heart for a fraction of a second.[14]

For the surgeons, the wait was the longest of their lives – the wait to see if the transplanted organ would start to beat in the chest of another person.

Washkansky lay there, motionless.

And then, following what felt like an eternity, it came like a lightning strike – a rapid contraction and then the heart started to move. The clock read 5.52am on that Sunday when Denise Darvall's heart started beating in Louis Washkansky's body.

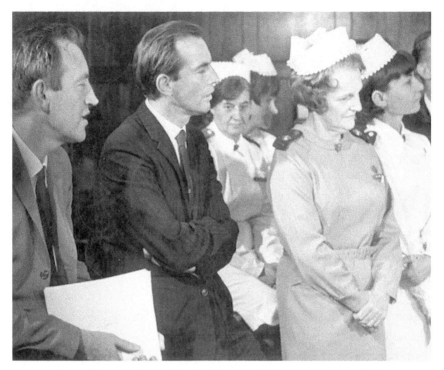

Some of the members of the first heart-transplantation team, including
(on the far left) Marius Barnard and Chris Barnard beside him.

PHOTOGRAPH COURTESY OF THE HEART OF CAPE TOWN MUSEUM

The last challenge was to see if the heart would continue to beat once Washkansky was taken off bypass. This happened slowly. And when Washy was weaned off the machine, the surgeons saw the new heart kick in.

Then Christiaan shouted: 'It's going to work!'

Someone started laughing. Someone else was cheering. The surgeons stood back. Time stood still for a moment when the new heart took over.

The efficacy of the new heart was analysed by the blood-pressure readings. Ozzy the anaesthesiologist read the blood-pressure readings aloud in one minute intervals amidst the new tension: 70 over 50, 75 over 50.[15] Slowly it crept up until, half an hour later, it was 100 over 80. The atmosphere in the theatre was celebratory.

Chris Barnard removed his surgical gloves and stated that he needed a cup of tea. On his way to the door, one sister hugged him spontaneously.

Five minutes later he was back and asking for updates on the blood-pressure readings. Shortly after this he stated that it was one of the greatest moments in medicine and he was proud.[16]

Still it wasn't over. The team had to ensure there were no leakages around the stitches. Then the chest had to be closed.

At 8.30am, Washkansky was finally wheeled to his specially prepared and sterilised room in Ward C2.[16] It was Sunday morning, 3 December 1967.

Anne Washkansky and Edward Darvall

Anne Washkansky received a call before midnight.

'Louis was already in the theatre. I stayed at home waiting for news. I phoned every hour. I phoned again at 6.00am and was told the operation had been a success. I asked Prof Barnard if the heart was working and he replied "beautifully". I wanted to cry.'

Barnard cautioned Anne that the next few days would be critical.

Edward Darvall, who had lost both his wife and his daughter, was in deep shock after the operation and was under sedation at his home in Tamboerskloof.

Stephen Darvall heard that his sister's heart had been transplanted only the next day on the radio.[17] Her kidney was also successfully transplanted, into the body of 10-year-old Jonathan van Wyk.

'My father didn't tell us everything,' Stephen Darvall recounted years later in an interview with *Die Burger*.[18] 'Many people said she had lived. She hadn't. She was young, 25. My mother was still young too.'

Johannes Barnard later commented on the irony of Christiaan doing the heart transplant on a Sunday morning.

'It was done at more or less the same time of the morning – and a Sunday, at that – that our father would set aside for his morning prayers.'[19]

For Christiaan, his father Adam was also uppermost in mind.

'When I sat in my car, there were tears of thankfulness in my eyes as I drove back to Zeekoevlei and I prayed to God and thanked him for giving me the opportunity to do this operation to the best of my ability. My father had always been so proud of his boys and I asked God to tell him what we had done to save a life.'[20]

The media storm started that same Sunday when informants at Groote Schuur leaked the news about the operation to the press.

Pamela Diamond, a journalist with the *Cape Times*, had known about the operation by midnight on Saturday. She spent Sunday trying to convince the on-duty news editor about the importance of the story – to no avail – and eventually drove to her editor's house to elicit his support in breaking the story on the front page.

Harry Shaw, a journalist for *Die Burger*, was woken up by a telephone call at around 5.25am on Sunday with the news. He and his colleagues worked throughout the day to break the story on the front page. At about midnight on the Sunday evening, when he had finished up and left the office, he walked into Marius Barnard and MC Botha, who had gone to the Naspers building with the news.

'Do you know about the heart transplant?' the doctors asked.

'Yes! And in a quarter of an hour, the printing press will be kicking in and you can read all about it in the paper tomorrow!' was Shaw's response.

CHAPTER 9

The man with the golden hands

L OUIS WASHKANSKY WOKE UP SMILING. HE COULDN'T SPEAK YET DUE TO
the tubes in his nose and throat. But he was smiling. And alive.

Later, when he was able speak, he was asked, 'Do you know where you
are?'

'Yes, I know. I'm in Groote Schuur Hospital. They promised me a new
heart. I feel a lot better now,' he said.[1]

There were endless questions for Christiaan Barnard too.

In archive footage, a French journalist with a thick black moustache
asked the last question of the press conference. He was standing to the
left of Barnard in the lecture room. The room was jam-packed.

'Doctor, will Mr Washkansky now have a long and healthy life?'

Barnard combed through his long straight hair with his fingers as he
leaned backwards in his chair before answering.

'It's always difficult making a prognosis about something that's never
been done before. I'm sure he will live longer than he would have done
without the operation. I cannot say how many months or days, but
there's no doubt that not only will he live longer, he will also be much
more comfortable than he was before.'[2]

There was not a single photograph taken of the Washkansky operation. The transplant team didn't think the operation would attract the
tremendous amounts of attention that it did.

'We were offered US$1 million for a photo of the donor heart in Louis'
chest, but there was none. We all knew it would be the first operation
ever and we expected it would make the news on the radio, but we never

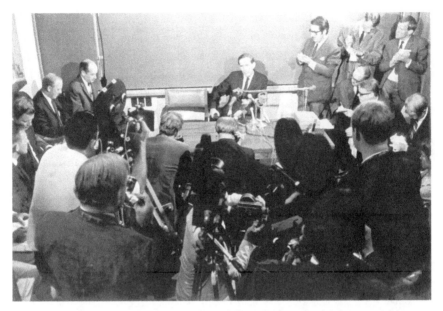

The media storm that hit Groote Schuur following the transplantation was like a tidal wave. The hospital and the team were wholly unprepared for the attention that they had unleashed. It was a situation similar to the lunar landing. Here Barnard is seated in a lecture room addressing the press.

PHOTOGRAPH COURTESY OF THE HEART OF CAPE TOWN MUSEUM

predicted the media storm that broke out. The fact that the transplant was done in Africa and not in the USA or Europe, came as a total shock to the world, especially once the journalists saw the young, unsophisticated doctors who had done the operation. Many people from across the world couldn't believe there was such a specialised hospital like Groote Schuur in Africa,' Marius Barnard recounts.[3]

Groote Schuur was inundated with messages of congratulations and support. The telegrams started flooding in.[4]

'Dear Chris, congratulations to you and your team on a fantastic achievement,' wrote Walton Lillehei.

Wangensteen's message said, 'Warm congratulations.'

American surgeons also praised Wangensteen for his ex-student's achievement, to which he replied, 'It's always nice to be praised for the achievements of your students. Chris Barnard was an exceptional chap. Chris Barnard is truly a phenomenon.'[5]

From New York, Adrian Kantrowitz suppressed his disappointment at not being first and said, 'Congratulations to you and your team on a magnificent achievement.'

Barnard's friends behind the Iron Curtain also celebrated his success. Prof Kolesnikov wrote, 'My warmest congratulations on your great success. Your deed will remain in history.'

A note that stands out is from Norman Shumway, the man who was at the forefront of heart-transplantation research and who had now been pipped to the post by Barnard.[6]

Shumway sent a longer message on 4 December, which can still be read at the Heart of Cape Town Museum. In the note Shumway wrote: 'Dear Chris, we read with fantastic interest your accomplishment of last Sunday evening. I am confident that DeBakey and Kantrowitz will not be far behind. From the reports in our newspapers, I would judge that you did a remarkable job synchronizing the ingredients of success for a heart transplant.'

Then Shumway, based on all his years of research into rejection, graciously also proffered some advice: 'Be certain to watch the R-wave of the ECG during the next several weeks for indices of rejection. It appears to be the earliest herald of important graft invasion.'

Shumway ended by stating, 'Everyone in the medical community wishes you success and compliments you and your team on a most significant event.'

Dr Lapa Munnik, a member of the provincial government and in charge of health services in the Cape Province, sent the team a telegram saying, 'Congratulations on the surgical Sputnik!'[7] Munnik told the Cape Times that the transplantation was a 'magnificent achievement'.

'One has always been aware that our medical research is equal to any in the world. I am proud that the first heart transplantation was done in South Africa.'

Sir Ray Hoffenberg was a specialist who started his career at Groote Schuur but went into exile in 1968 following his anti-apartheid activities.

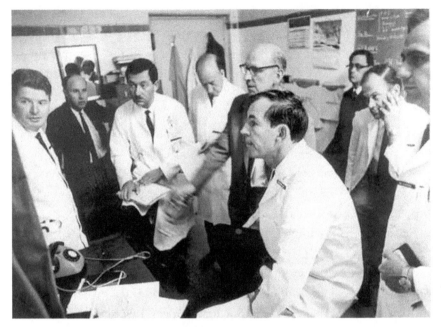

Following the successful transplantation, the Groote Schuur team monitored Louis Washkansky's condition closely. Pictured here in the 'war room' are Chris Barnard, (behind him) Bossie Bosman, and MC Botha (at the back wearing glasses). The team hardly slept in the weeks following the transplant.

PHOTOGRAPH COURTESY OF THE HEART OF CAPE TOWN MUSEUM

He wrote later that Barnard's success was praised for being a miracle.

'For the South African government, amidst huge criticism and threats of being rejected from the global village, the operation was a godsend. Could things really be that bad in a country where such an outstanding first in medicine was achieved?'

It wasn't only the medical fraternity and the government that was raving about the operation. Thousands of letters and messages kept streaming into Groote Schuur from the public. They were mostly very flattering, but some accused Barnard and the Groote Schuur team of performing pseudoscience and being ungodly.

One letter writer addressed Christiaan Barnard as 'The Butcher of

Groote Schuur' and stated that he was a 'human vulture'.

Others begged him to stop with the procedures on religious grounds. 'Man can't replace God's will.'

Still another wrote, 'It is my profound conviction you are unmoral. A bunch of ghouls, all of you.'

The controversy about putting one person's heart into another rapidly escalated. Well-known personalities such as the British TV host Malcolm Muggeridge stated that people considered heart transplants to be unnatural and that it was interfering with being human and trespassing in the realm of spirituality.

The Vatican's newspaper and mouthpiece for Roman Catholicism, *L'Osservatore Romano*, came out strongly in favour of Barnard's achievement. In an editorial, the newspaper stated that the world was getting too emotional over the successful heart transplant in South Africa.[8] In what was described as a philosophical editorial, the editor, Raimondo Manzini, said that the young woman whose heart had been used had simply provided a mechanical organ that was necessary for physical life, but didn't provide a life of its own.

'The emotional reaction is mainly due to humanity paying its respects to a young woman who died in the prime of her youth in a motor accident and gave her "dead heart" so that it could live again and provide life to another.'

The article went on to say that the heart was a physiological organ with a mechanical function. Human organs are physically part of the body but don't define humanity.[9]

Other letters from children included one from a 10-year-old schoolgirl, Sheri, who asked Barnard if he thought women could also become heart surgeons.

Other letters highlighted the controversies that were raging.

One young boy asked, 'If a doctor says you're dead and removes your heart but the heart is still beating, are you dead or alive?'

Barnard's team members were also thrust into the media spotlight. MC Botha became a firm favourite.

'The first question everyone asks me is if we can do the tissue testing. They simply cannot believe that we could determine all the factors here in Cape Town; they cannot even do it in England. Then they want to know how it's possible that we can do it here. My answer is just to laugh and say, "well, we did do it here."'[10]

The American surgeon James Hardy, who had placed the heart of a chimpanzee into a human three years earlier was very disappointed when he heard about the success in Cape Town. He was sorry that he had not taken his work further.

'I was attending a Christmas party when someone told me about the operation in South Africa. My evening was spoiled. We should have done it. But given the position I was in following that first transplant, my decision taken at the time was the correct one. Still, I am sorry I had to have taken that decision.'[11]

The second heart transplant

Three days after the first historic heart transplant in Cape Town, the world's second transplant was done, this time in Brooklyn, New York.[12] The surgeon was Adrian Kantrowitz and his patient was Jamie Scudero, a two-and-a-half-week-old baby boy. The 22-member medical team worked for two hours and 15 minutes to save the baby's life with a heart transplant.

'We were trying to make one whole individual from two individuals who stood no chance of survival when they were born,' Kantrowitz said.[13]

Scudero survived six-and-a-half hours with his new heart before he died.[14]

The preparations for this surgery had begun a week before the Washkansky operation. A donor heart was found after more than 500 telegrams were sent to American hospitals seeking help for Scudero. The donor was an anencephalic baby, one born without a large part of its brain. Anencephalic babies survive for, at best, three days.[15]

Kantrowitz and his Brooklyn team had been ready to do a heart transplant 18 months earlier following his intensive research during which he'd experimented on more than 250 dogs.[16]

On 29 June 1966 – 18 months before the Groote Schuur transplant – Kantrowitz was prevented from doing the world's first human-to-human transplant on a baby. The donor's parents had provided permission and the surgeons were seconds away from proceeding when two older and more senior hospital staff stopped the proceedings. The chief paediatrician and anaesthetist argued at the time that Kantrowitz couldn't continue while the donor's heart was still beating.[17] By the time the tiny heart stopped beating, it was too late as it rapidly degenerated.

Then, on 2 December 1967, as Kantrowitz was yet again poised to perform the first operation, his daughter woke him up with the news that a man called Barnard had beaten him to it.

'You can't always be first. Some races you lose, others you win.'[18]

Three days later, the American performed the world's second heart transplant.

There was good reason to believe that babies would fare better with organ transplantation than adults. People are born with hardly any immune system. This starts to develop fully from six months. In the interim, babies are protected by the antibodies they receive from their mothers' breastmilk, especially from the colostrum they get immediately after birth. Accordingly, any blood type could be put into a baby without complications, but do the same with adults and the reaction could lead to death. It was believed that the same would be the case for organ transplantation. The chance was that organs would not be rejected if transplanted at a young age, before the body's immune system was fully in place.

Following the death of Kantrowitz's patient, Barnard expressed his condolences and stated that the operation on a tiny baby would have been much more difficult than on Washkansky.[19]

Kantrowitz became the first American to perform a human-to-human heart transplant, thereby beating the more established and more experienced Shumway and Lower.[20]

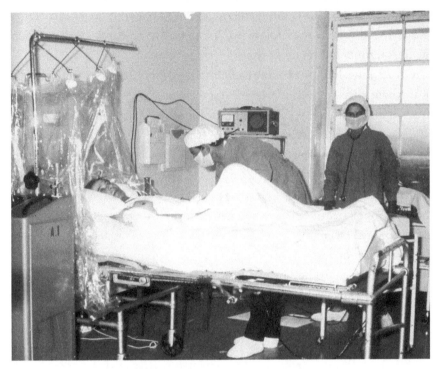

*Chris Barnard tending to Louis Washkansky with Sister
Georgie de Klerk in the background.*

PHOTOGRAPH COURTESY OF THE HEART OF CAPE TOWN MUSEUM

In Cape Town, the 53-year-old Washkansky was showing signs of a person with a will to live. Anne wasn't allowed to visit her husband for the first few days due to the risk of infection.

'I'm not prepared to put my husband in danger; he's too precious to me to simply storm in there,' she said in the media.

The media were having a field day and compared the heart transplant in Cape Town to the greatest human achievements ever.

Time magazine's headline on 15 December 1967 stated, 'The Ultimate Operation' with one subtitle reading, 'Equal to Everest'.

On 18 December, *Newsweek* led with 'The Heart: Miracle in Cape Town'.

The man with the golden hands

The 50-year-old television imagery is in black and white and shaky, because the person holding the camera was a doctor, not an experienced cameraman. This was the only way Barnard would allow any footage to be taken of Washkansky inside his sterile room. In the footage, Louis Washkansky sits upright in his bed and smiles. This was only a few days after the epic operation.

'I was lucky enough to get a second chance. Very few people do.'[21]

On 7 December, the South African state broadcaster, the SABC, did a live radio interview with Washkansky. Bossie Bosman was the interviewer.

Bosman: 'And how are you feeling, Mr Washkansky?'

Washkansky: 'I'm feeling good.'

Bosman: 'Are you feeling healthy?'

Washkansky: 'Yes, quite fine.'

Bosman: 'What would you like to eat tonight?'

Washkansky: 'Something light.'

Bosman: 'How does it feel to be such a famous man?'

Washkansky: 'I'm not famous. The doctor's famous – the man with the golden hands.'

That afternoon Anne Washkansky was reunited with her husband for the first time. She told him how famous he was; his name was even in lights on the big Sanlam building in the centre of Cape Town.

'What have I done? I did nothing,' Washkansky said.

When she left, her husband told her how happy he was to have seen her. 'Good-bye, kid,' he said.

Louis Washkansky started the second week of his second life by asking for a steak and a cold beer – a request that was turned down by his doctors.

The old streetfighter who refused to give up improved rapidly with most of his symptoms clearing up as his new heart flushed his body with richly oxygenated blood. His sense of humour, which had been absent for months, returned and Washy started calling the assistant who regularly took blood samples, 'Old Dracula'.[22] He also referred to himself as the new Frankenstein.

Washkansky was pumped full of drugs daily in an effort to combat rejection but his condition kept improving and soon he was starting to make plans to return home for Christmas, a few weeks away.[23]

On 10 December, *Cape Times* journalist John Scott wrote on the front page about the post-operative period that Washkansky was entering. He explained that it was the most dangerous period for the patient.

'The danger that the organ could be rejected by his body is imminent. Two factors make him very susceptible to infection, the medicine he is given to combat rejection and his diabetes.'

In addition, radiation treatment was destroying valuable white blood cells. This combination would expose Washkansky's body to infection because its defences were being suppressed.

Scott would become the first journalist in the *Cape Times*'s history to have his name published next to his stories following his investigative journalism on the heart transplant.

On the 10th day after the transplant, Washkansky walked a few steps and sat in the sun on the balcony, the first time in months that he had tasted the outdoors.[24] Anne kept visiting and remarked how Louis was looking better than he had in two years. Her old Louis from before his heart disease was making a comeback.

The couple's 14-year-old son, Michael, and other family members also visited, as well as Solly Sklar, of course. Solly joked about the party they would throw when Washkansky came home.

It was probably all too good to be true.

Despite the very best efforts of the Barnard team – some staff were on duty for 24-hour intervals – 12 days after the transplant, there was a downturn and Washkansky started to complain of chest pain. He also developed a fever.

Washkansky started coughing up phlegm and X-rays showed a shadow on the lungs. The Groote Schuur doctors diagnosed the problem as pneumonia and decided that immediate treatment was needed. The team went into overdrive to address the new threat and he was given a strong dose of penicillin over a 24-hour period.[25]

Washkansky didn't improve; in fact, his white blood cell count started to plummet. As is the case after most big operations, his white blood cell count had been up to three times the normal but now the numbers had fallen alarmingly within a few hours to a new low level.

To tackle the situation, haematologists infused eight litres of blood. Then another 25 billion white blood cells were injected into Washkansky's veins. Still his white blood count didn't increase and the destruction of his body's cells continued.[26] Finally, 18 days after Louis Washkansky got his new heart, he died.

The post-mortem was done immediately. The only good news was that his death was not related to the new heart. The courageous man had died of double pneumonia, but the heart of Denise Darvall had remained strong and healthy all the way to the end.

This was nevertheless a blow to all.

Anne Washkansky, however, was satisfied. She knew that her husband had died a happy man.

'He kept fighting to the end. For 18 days longer, the doctors gave him hope and a new belief and faith. In these 18 days, Prof Barnard gave me back my old Louis, even if it was for a few days. The old Louis with whom I had fallen in love and married. The Louis filled with enthusiasm and jokes.'

Louis was dead but Anne would take away many bittersweet memories.

'My 21 years with Louis were worth more to me than 50 years with anyone else,' the newly widowed woman said.[27]

The media storm hit a new frenzy.

A journalist from *Die Burger*, Harry Shaw, got one of the few scoops at this time when he managed to get hold of a copy of the cardiogram showing Washkansky's last heartbeats.

'I worked my contacts hard. One phoned and offered the cardiogram in exchange for a new Leica camera. I agreed. The cardiogram was published on the front page and attracted a lot of attention. Dr Barnard was set to go to America later that day and held a press conference first. His colleagues showed him the cardiogram and he was furious and wanted it returned immediately.

'Barnard thought we'd stolen it but that was impossible. The contact got such a fright, he informed me he wasn't interested in the Leica camera any longer.'

On the day Louis died, the media asked Christiaan Barnard if the death of the patient negated in any way the success of the 'experiment'.

Barnard's reply was simple: 'I don't like to refer to heart transplantation as an experiment. This was a clinical treatment of a sick patient. Although Mr Washkansky is dead, I don't believe we have any evidence that suggests heart transplantation for certain cardiological diseases is not a good idea.'[28]

Still, Washkansky's death raised questions about performing heart transplantation.

'Should heart transplantation be done at this early stage, especially when the rejection problem has not yet been resolved?'[29]

The criticism was surprising given that kidney and liver transplants had already been done for some time, despite the ongoing lack of clarity around rejection.

One member of the heart team simply said, 'We climbed Everest. Next time we'll know how to come down again.'[30]

At this stage, the 10-year-old Jonathan van Wyk who had received Denise Darvall's kidney, was still in a stable condition in Karl Bremer Hospital in Bellville.

Reacting to the death of Washkansky, Kantrowitz stated that, despite his own failure two weeks earlier, he still believed that the first operation by Barnard had been a giant step forward.[31]

Washkansky was buried in Pinelands Jewish Cemetery on the day after he died. The transplant team were asked to be coffin bearers. Christiaan Barnard turned the request down, stating that it would create a media circus for the family that was best avoided.[32] However, MC Botha and Marius Barnard agreed to represent the hospital.

Edward Darvall never recovered from the trauma of the accident and was unable to sleep again without sleeping pills.[33]

'He was devastated. The accident destroyed him and he never went to work again. Twenty-seven months later, Edward Darvall was also dead, leaving behind two young boys to fend for themselves.

After a stint doing national service, Stephen Darvall cared for his younger brother.

'That's life. You can't change it. A person never thinks something like this will happen to you,' Stephen said to *Die Burger* later.

Stephen met Barnard once.

'Dr Barnard looked like a decent enough man. I met him once in 1968 at City Hall. Today, though, most people don't even recognise the name. People forget. And it's almost 50 years ago.'

PART THREE

The global doctor, 1968–1983

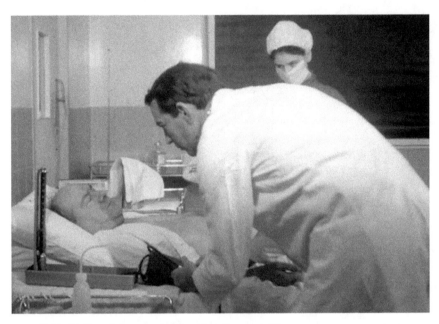

Philip Blaiberg being checked by Chris Barnard. 'He was not an easy patient.
He let you know he was a doctor,' recalls Sister Georgie de Klerk,
who tended to Washkansky and Blaiberg.

CHAPTER 10

Blaiberg

DAYS AFTER WASHKANSKY'S FUNERAL, CHRISTIAAN BARNARD WENT on a whirlwind tour of Europe and America where he spoke on the miracle operation in Cape Town. Louwtjie went with him.

The couple first went to Washington DC, where Barnard appeared on television on 24 December 1967 with his American counterparts, Kantrowitz and DeBakey.

Barnard stated that, despite the death of Washkansky, heart transplantation showed great promise in providing an alternative for hundreds of thousands of patients with incurable heart disease who were staring an inevitable death in the face.

Kantrowitz agreed that the world had entered a new era, while DeBakey said he, too, shared the enthusiasm about transplantation representing a 'great step forward'. The three surgeons also agreed that rejection remained the greatest challenge when it came to heart transplantation.

The Barnards spent Christmas in New York, far from friends and family. For Christiaan, it was a wonderful time and totally different from his first experiences of America.

In 1955, he had had to shovel snow to buy food. This time around, he was given first-class treatment all the way and became the centre of attention in the city that never sleeps.

For Louwtjie, however, this was her first bad experience with the fame that her husband had attracted. Louwtjie's husband was shaking hands all over the Big Apple while she remained in the hotel room.

'We stayed in a suite at the Plaza Hotel. It had a wonderful view over Central Park. It was bitterly cold. Through the windows I could see children ice-skating. That day I was sad for the first time. It was the first time I was away from my home and my children for Christmas and there was nobody to say Merry Christmas to. There wasn't even a Christmas card from my husband.'[1]

Christiaan's old mentor and friend, Walton Lillehei, happened to be in New York at the time and the two spent some time together.

'I had not been surprised when I got the news on 3 December, hearing surgeons in Cape Town had done the transplant. I knew immediately who it was.'[2]

Lillehei said that both Shumway and Kantrowitz had been ready to go ahead and do the operation first, but the Americans were impeded by the problem of when the donors are legally dead. Brain death was still not an acceptable measure of clinical death in the United States at the time.

'Conversations with Shumway indicated that he believed the public would not be happy if a donor's heart was removed from a living donor before it had stopped beating. It took great courage from Chris to go ahead and do the operation,' said Lillehei.[3]

In New York, the two surgeons paid a visit to the newly appointed South African Consul to the United Nations, Pik Botha.

'I was invited to go along with Chris to visit him. He had never met Chris before. I remember he said, "Dr Barnard, thank you for everything you are doing for your country. Most people think we South Africans live in mud huts and wear grass skirts and are quite primitive,"' Lilllehei recalls.[4]

Walton Lillehei

Lillehei's life story is as colourful as that of Christiaan Barnard's. Despite his remarkable efforts and pioneering work in Minneapolis, he was passed over for promotion when Wangensteen retired. He resigned and moved to New York, initially going without his family. When he left Minnesota, he took along all his laboratory equipment, moving it all out one Sunday and leaving behind nothing but a red rose in the centre of the room. In New York, Lillehei developed a reputation as a womaniser and party animal, before he eventually lost his job at the age of 51.

Then the taxman went after him. Lillehei had not paid any taxes for many years and in 1972 a jury indicted him on charges of tax evasion amounting to US$125 100. Lillehei was facing a 25-year jail term on the charges. Part of the investigation by the IRS revealed a secret life of mistresses, including Las Vegas call girls. The jury found Lillehei guilty on all counts but the judge couldn't bring himself to destroy a man with Lillehei's abilities. Instead of jail time, Lillehei was fined $50 000 and given six months' community service. At the age of 55, Lillehei stopped performing surgery and started the process of rehabilitation. The medical fraternity eventually welcomed him back into the fold.[5]

Despite her misgivings, Louwtjie tried to enjoy the experience and recognised that she was part of something special.

'I often told myself, "Woman, enjoy every moment, this experience only comes along once in a person's life." The big hotel cupboards with our little bits of luggage, however, eventually looked so empty.'[6]

At the end of the tour, the Barnards went to Texas to visit the American President, Lyndon Johnson.

'His farm was just a plain old farm. The only difference was the armed guards. His wife was very friendly and a lovely person, very pretty. Her first words were, 'Hi folks! Welcome to America!'' Louwtjie recalled.[7]

'I was at ease. The president and his wife were normal people. He was huge and well built. I felt like a dwarf but they were friendly. Chris and the president initially spoke about the heart transplantation and later about farming. Our visit was initially meant to be half an hour but it lasted more than four hours after they invited us to lunch.'

Johnson took Barnard in a helicopter across his farm, the first time the Karoo boy had been in one.

'It looked like there was more wildlife on that farm than in the Kruger Park,' Barnard said.[8]

The following day the couple returned to South Africa.

Philip Blaiberg

On his return to Cape Town, Christiaan Barnard would perform his second heart transplant, Dr Philip Blaiberg, a 58-year-old retired dentist from Cape Town.[9] He had been forced to retire at a young age due to his heart condition.

By December 1967, Blaiberg was dying and he knew it. For years he had been struggling to breathe and had had to rely on machines at times for oxygen. His bodily functions were already severely affected by the heart disease.[10]

'Death would have been a welcome release,' Blaiberg stated.[11]

His trouble had started 14 years earlier, when he and his son were climbing Lion's Head, a peak alongside Table Mountain.

'I felt a sharp pain in my chest and decided to leave the climbing and return home instead.'

Two weeks later Blaiberg had a heart attack and became a patient of Velva Schrire's, whom he said 'saved my life'. Following intensive treatment, Blaiberg was placed on a healthy diet and given strong heart medication. This enabled him to live the next few years in relative comfort, but with a sword hanging over his head.

'In January 1967, things changed. I was exhausted at work. It was difficult to get up in the mornings.'

On Sunday 5 March 1967, Blaiberg had a second heart attack and believed he was dying. He was rushed to hospital, where Schrire attended to him. Schrire told Blaiberg's wife, Eileen, that her husband's days were numbered.

'He said, besides a new heart, there was nothing else that could help or save Phil,' she said.

The dentist stopped working permanently to rest at home. From

September 1967, Blaiberg was more in bed than out of it and he became increasingly weak and depressed.[12]

'This continued until 3 December, when I heard about the heart transplant on the radio.'

From that moment, Blaiberg wouldn't stop talking about a heart transplant. Eileen contacted Schrire, who informed her that he had, in fact, already put forward Blaiberg's name as a candidate for a heart transplant.

'Prof Schrire said Phil was next on the list. Suddenly there was hope.'

Eileen asked her husband how he'd feel about the chance to get a new heart.

'He stretched out his arms and said, "The sooner the better". He made me promise that no matter the outcome of Washkansky's transplant, I would stand by him all the way. There we were, two adults, married more than 30 years and laughing and crying like children.'[13]

Blaiberg was smuggled into Groote Schuur Hospital on 16 December 1967, a public holiday.

'The place was a madhouse following the Washkansky operation. In addition, the news had leaked to the media that a second transplant was on the way. Then my name was leaked, despite our best efforts to keep it secret,' says Blaiberg.

The cat was out the bag and the media had a new obsession.

Blaiberg first met Christiaan Barnard on 17 December, when he repeated his willingness to go ahead with a transplant – the sooner the better.

'I was satisfied. Here was a man in whose hands I would willingly place my life. I learnt to know him well and know he has a determined personality and is utterly dedicated to his craft,' said Blaiberg.

The excitement lasted until 21 December – the morning that Louis Washkansky died.

'I was surprised to see my wife early that morning. She used to come visit in the afternoon. Shortly after her arrival, Prof Barnard arrived,' Blaiberg recalls.

For Eileen, Washkansky's death came as a great shock just as she was starting to believe in the operation. She wanted to leave the room but Barnard asked her to stay.[14]

'Barnard looked tired, no longer like the handsome Jan Smuts but more like the martyred Christ. Something had happened to dampen the optimism and the spring in his step,' Blaiberg said.

Barnard started off, 'I feel like a pilot who has crashed his plane.' Blaiberg still didn't know what was going on. Then Barnard asked him if he knew that Washkansky had died that morning; that he had died of pneumonia. Blaiberg suddenly understood why the two of them were so upset.

Barnard continued, 'To be honest, we did the first one and the patient has now died. But we think we learnt a lot and we can still offer you something.'

Without hesitation, Blaiberg said, 'When can you operate?'

I want to continue now more than ever before, not only for my benefit but also for yours and all those people who did so much to try and save Louis Washkansky.'

Blaiberg's decision was final. Nothing could dissuade him. A new heart was his only chance at survival and he grabbed it without hesitation.[15]

Clive Haupt

Cape Town. New Year's Day, 1968. The entire city was on holiday.

The 24-year-old Clive Haupt had been looking forward to the New Year's Day festivities. He was one of 11 children of a coloured family who had been raised in a two-bedroomed home in Athlone.[16] He had left school after Standard 6 because his mother, Muriel, could no longer afford to keep him in school. His father was dead by this time.

At 16 years old, Clive started work in a factory that made breakfast cereal. Three years later, he got a job as a machinist in a clothing factory. There he met Dorothy Snyders.

The pair shared many interests and enjoyed spending time together, often going to the cinema or playing card games at home. After they had been dating for a year, the couple got married in St Luke's Anglican Church on 13 August 1966, Dorothy's birthday. The Haupts moved into a home in Portland Street in Salt River.

Clive and his young wife were looking forward to celebrating the New Year together with their friends. It started out well, with a wonderful time on the beach at Glencairn between Muizenberg and Simon's Town. They had all met up at about 9.00am and were enjoying themselves.[17]

At about 2.00pm they started a ball game. Clive played while Dorothy watched.[18] Suddenly he made a playful dive onto Dorothy and fell on the beach in front of her, where he remained, unmoving.

While many of the bystanders thought Clive was play-acting, Dorothy quickly realised that something was seriously wrong. Foam was coming out of her husband's mouth. He was already unconscious.

The crowd reacted swiftly and Clive was rushed to the closest hospital in False Bay. From there an ambulance took him to the larger Victoria Hospital in Wynberg, which had better facilities.[19]

Clive had been struck down by a brain haemorrhage and he was in critical condition. A doctor at Victoria Hospital phoned Groote Schuur and an ambulance was sent to fetch Clive. Dorothy and her aunt went along in the ambulance.[20]

At around 5.00pm Clive Haupt arrived at Groote Schuur Hospital and was admitted to Ward C-2, where every effort was made to save his life.[21]

This is where Ray Hoffenberg came into the picture. By this time, he was known for being an ardent anti-apartheid activist and had angered the government no end. He had been charged under the Suppression of Communism Act, which was going to prevent him from working at any institution of learning in the country. This banning order was to kick in the following day.

Haupt was the last patient Hoffenberg admitted in South Africa. He and his wife left the country on a one-way exit visa shortly afterwards.

'On my last night as a consultant on duty, the transplant team asked me to declare a young man dead and to confirm his heart was in an acceptable shape for a transplant.'[22]

Hoffenberg initially refused to declare Haupt dead and insisted on further treatment.

Throughout the night, Coert Venter discussed the situation with Dorothy and Muriel, Clive's mother, and asked whether, were Clive to be declared dead, they could have permission to transplant his heart into the body of someone who was dying. Muriel said that if this were the case and they could save another life, they could use her son's heart.

Clive stayed alive through the night – connected to machines – but by morning he was rapidly deteriorating.

In the hallway at the hospital, Eileen Blaiberg had seen the Haupt family in passing.

'They were waiting on news about Clive. Phil was in the meantime still unaware of what was going on and was angry because his pills and water had been taken away already. Then when they said the operation was on the way, he became excited. He surprised me. No-one would have believed he was about to undergo the most complicated and difficult operation imaginable.'

'Finally,' Blaiberg said. 'Finally, you bastards are going to do something!'

The entire transplant team was called in again at 9.10am. Christiaan Barnard arrived at 9.30am. His brother Marius and MC Botha were already there.

Hoffenberg finally declared Haupt dead at 10.42am after no reflexes were found. At 11.00am on Tuesday, 2 January 1968, the world's third heart transplantation started.

Outside Groote Schuur the media circus was getting frenetic. The world wanted to see Barnard and his team in action and the news was out that the operation was proceeding.

Inside the theatre the procedure proved to be very challenging. The heart-lung machine broke down at one stage when one of the tubes broke. The result was that the theatre was sprayed with blood before cool heads prevailed and the machine was rapidly repaired by the technician, Johan van Heerden.[23]

In addition, Barnard was struggling with a severe flare-up of his arthritis. In an article entitled 'Miracle Man' published in July 1968 in the *Orange Coast Magazine*, Barnard described how he had struggled to do the operation with his affliction causing him immense agony and problems. He said that the attack was one of the worst arthritic flare-ups he had ever had.

The disease is made worse by periods of high emotional and physical stress.

After all the excitement of the first transplant and the accompanying and exhausting tour overseas, Barnard had walked straight into the theatre to work on Blaiberg. He was in such agony that an assistant had to help him prepare for the surgery.

'My hands and fingers were stiff and painful, it was especially bad when I had to do the sutures.'[24]

Despite these challenges, the world's third transplant was another huge success for Barnard and Groote Schuur.

Racial controversy

At 3.45pm, a member of the medical team walked out of the theatre and announced to the gathered media that Blaiberg's new heart had started to beat.[25]

The following day, a race controversy developed when it became known that a white dentist had received the heart of a coloured man.

Media houses across the globe latched onto the issue. The British *Guardian* wrote in a report entitled 'Brothers Under the Skin' that in South Africa, not even blood transfusions between races were allowed under apartheid legislation, but now Blaiberg owed his life to a coloured man.

Another paper wanted to know if Blaiberg would still be classified 'white' since his heart was no longer the heart of a white man.

The controversy was considered to be ironic given that the media had not said a word about the fact that Darvall's kidney had been transplanted into a coloured boy, Jonathan van Wyk, a month earlier.

The race issue would continue for years.

Five days after the operation, Blaiberg was already recovering well.

'I was alive, and I could breathe without effort or coughing. People asked me if I felt different with someone else's heart in my body. I never once felt different; I'm still the old Philip Blaiberg. I'm still just as fond of Italian food and red wine.'[26]

Blaiberg became a huge success story for Groote Schuur. He lived for a further 19 months and 15 days.

Eileen Blaiberg attended the funeral of Clive Haupt. It was one of the biggest funerals ever held in Cape Town, with an estimated 6 000 mourners joining Eileen at the Woltemade Cemetery in Maitland.

The secret heart photographs

Philip Blaiberg's heart transplant, the world's third, served up a drama that would not have been out of place in a James Bond thriller.

The world was obsessed with heart transplantation following the Washkansky breakthrough and the demand for photographs of a heart transplant being done reached dizzying heights.

In a time before the lunar landing, this was a global event considered to be on a par with the conquering of Everest.

There were no photographs of the Washkansky operation. The Groote Schuur team simply never considered that it might turn out to be as significant as it did.

The world's second heart transplantation was done on a six-day-old baby who died within hours. There were no photographs of that either.

The pressure was on for that first exclusive photograph of a human heart transplantation and if this could include a picture of the miracle man – Chris Barnard – in action, the journalist who supplied it knew they would be guaranteed a giant pay cheque.

The media frenzy outside Groote Schuur Hospital through December 1967 into January 1968, following the Washkansky operation, was incredible. The tension was palpable as the world's media outlets waited for Barnard to do another heart transplant.

Around 150 of the world's best and most experienced newshounds were permanently staking out the hospital following rumours of a second patient – a dentist called Blaiberg – inside, waiting for a donor. All these journalists were trying to get that exclusive image.

The chance of getting it, however, was zero. Groote Schuur had been secured by all means possible, including permanent police and security guards, even inside the hospital.

Journalists were caught trying to sneak in dressed as nurses, and climbing trees and lamp posts to get photographs of Blaiberg, all to no avail.

Rumours started circulating of an American television network having secured exclusive rights to film the next operation. In addition, it was said that Barnard's friend, the photographer Don Mackenzie, would also take photographs of the historic operation.

As it turned out, the Blaibergs had concluded an exclusive deal with NBC, allowing the American television network to film the operation for US$50 000.

Mackenzie was denied permission to attend the operation and he left the hospital early in the day.

When NBC's film crews arrived for the operation, they were chased away by Barnard, who couldn't allow the risk of infection in the theatre. One producer for NBC stated at the time, 'The operation took place so fast, no-one filmed.'

Accordingly, there was no-one inside the theatre to film or take photographs of the third-ever heart transplantation.

Or so everyone believed.

Two freelance photographers from Cape Town managed to achieve what all the rest could not.

In the weeks before the operation, Sigurd Olivier and Brian Astbury developed a contact on Barnard's extended heart-transplantation team, who agreed to take sneak photographs of the Blaiberg operation.[27]

Dr Reuben Mibashan was a haematologist who had a small, indirect role during the operation that required him to be in the theatre. He was disgruntled because he felt that the heart-transplantation team was receiving more than its fair share of funding from the hospital, which was limiting his own department's research.

Olivier showed Mibashan his media credentials and told him that they would split the money 50/50.

'We could make R15 000 and you can use the money for your research,'

Olivier told Mibashan, who said that it would certainly help with his work.

The doctor had access to a tiny Minox 16mm spy camera and said he would use it to take the photographs during the operation.

'So our plans were made. Since no-one knew exactly when the operation would happen, Brian and I spent 24-hour shifts in my van outside the hospital. Our plan was simple. I would wait on the steps down the hall outside the theatre and Mibashan would bring me the camera after he took the photos. Brian and I would then have the photos developed and get them out on the wires once a deal had been struck,' Olivier recalls.

Forty minutes into the Blaiberg operation, things were going according to plan for the duo. Then Mibashan arrived, ashen-faced ,on the steps.

'What's wrong?' asked Olivier.

'I was seen,' Mibashan replied, the tiny camera in his hand.

Someone on the transplant team had seen him taking the photos.

'He said it would cost him his career. I felt sorry for the man and lacked the killer instinct, that other newshounds had perhaps [to pressure Hibashan], else we would have made a lot of money,' says Olivier.

Mibashan went on to say that there was no-one else in the theatre taking photos or filming the operation that was still in progress. The tiny film increased tenfold in value.

Olivier suggested that they develop the film before making any decisions. Mibashan agreed and handed over the film, which was swiftly developed into 6x4-inch photos, showing the Barnard team transplanting Blaiberg's heart.

The trio met again hours later and Mibashan was even more upset.

'He wanted us to wait till matters could be cleared up. So we gave him the film and a set of photos,' says Olivier.

Mibashan told the duo that a total embargo had been placed on the photographs by hospital authorities.

'Three months later, we were approached by a media outlet offering us R 120 000 for the photos – a lot of money in those days,' sighs Olivier.

Still Mibashan wouldn't budge.

Barnard was vaguely aware of what had been happening in his theatre.

'A senior member of the team smuggled in a camera. Without permission, Dr Mibashan quietly took some photos during the proceedings but was caught out. We were very shocked. I recall thinking it strange that a haematologist was so interested in this operation. The photos were of poor quality and were taken away from Mibashan [by Jannie Louw]. I never saw them again,' Chris Barnard recalled later.

'I also never saw Mibashan again; his career at the hospital came to a sudden end,' Barnard said.

Mibashan emigrated to England in 1970, where he continued to work as a medical lecturer and professor. He died in 2001.[27]

The original film and set of photos have long since disappeared. Probably only Jannie Louw, Groote Schuur head of surgery, ever knew what became of them.

What people didn't know, however, was that Olivier and Astbury had developed two sets of photos and held onto the one set. The original idea was to have a set of photographs to use in negotiations with media outlets.

This never transpired. Mibashan's position had placed the two media men in a difficult spot and they decided not to sell or publish the photos.

Until now.

The first photos ever taken of a heart transplantation being done, showing Chris Barnard in action, are published here with the permission of Olivier and Astbury.

Brian went on to found and run The Space in Cape Town, South Africa's first non-racial theatre, and Sigurd became a successful publisher. However, some of his books were banned in apartheid South Africa.

Brian now lives in London, while Sigurd lives in the Netherlands.

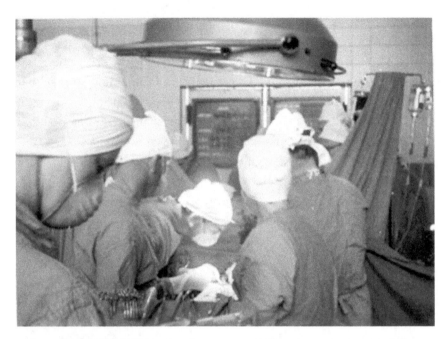

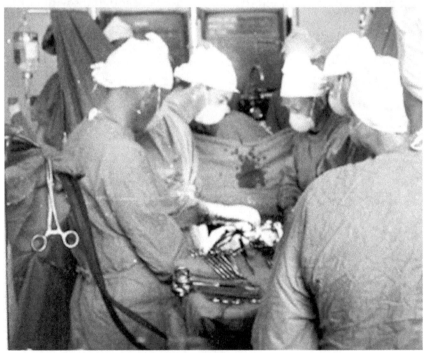

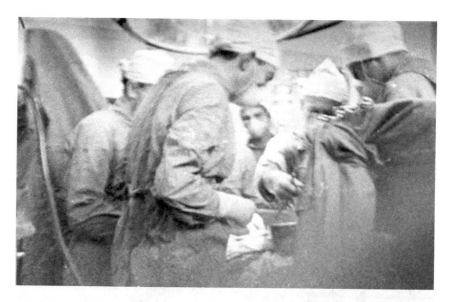

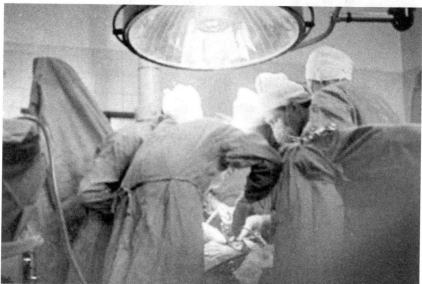

This sequence of photographs has never been published before and are the earliest known photographs of a heart transplantation being performed. Chris Barnard can be easily identified in action here. These pictures were taken with a 16mm spy camera during the Philip Blaiberg operation. The film was as small as a woman's pinkie nail.

PHOTOGRAPHS COURTESY OF SIGURD OLIVIER AND BRIAN ASTBURY

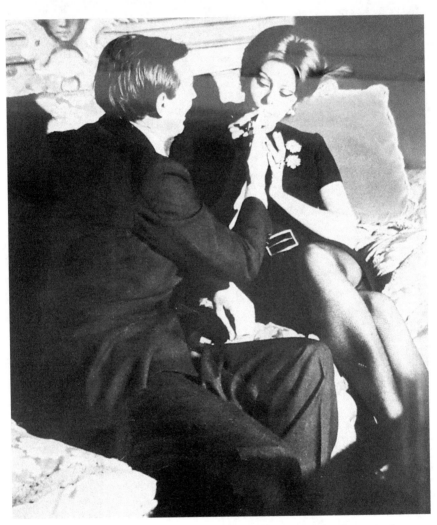

Chris Barnard became the darling of the world, considered to be a miracle worker. He developed a close bond with many famous actors and actresses including Sophia Loren, who in years to come, would often approach him for help with Italians, mainly children, who had heart problems.

PHOTOGRAPH COURTESY OF THE HEART OF CAPE TOWN MUSEUM

CHAPTER 11

Three women and the Pope

V IRGINIA WHITE AND HER HUSBAND CHARLES HAD BEEN HIGH SCHOOL sweethearts. On Thursday 4 January 1968 they celebrated their 22nd wedding anniversary. The following night the 43-year-old American computer programmer was struck down by a blood clot. By late evening there was nothing further doctors could do for her.[1]

Mrs White was an organ donor and her heart would make the world's fourth heart transplantation possible, on 6 January 1968. The patient was Mike Kasperak, a steelworker, and the surgeon was Norman Shumway.

At last the 44-year-old Shumway, head of the heart unit at Stanford University in Palo Alto, California, would get his chance to apply his hard-earned knowledge on a human being.

Shumway's first procedure received tremendous media attention. Journalists even scaled walls at the hospital trying to see into the operating theatre.[2]

The operation was a success, but Kasperak died 14 days later. He was simply too sick, with many other afflictions, and his body couldn't withstand the procedure.

Heart transplant surgeons in the early days received patients that were very ill. After all, doctors would not recommend a patient for such a daring operation unless there was no further hope and a new heart was their last chance.

By the time of their procedures, these patients were often quite weak and suffering from a range of complex problems, which could not be fixed by simply getting a new heart. Washkansky, for example, suffered from diabetes. These additional afflictions, which contributed to the deaths of most of the early transplant patients, often meant that the heart transplants were unfairly judged as unsuccessful.[3]

After his first heart transplant, Shumway noted that the procedure was easier on humans than it was on animals. In a rare comment on Barnard, Shumway also praised the South African for proving that a human body with a transplanted heart could be resuscitated and that a transplanted heart could work in another body.

'While the animal research indicated it could be possible, it wasn't proven before.'

Shumway's legacy

Shumway's early failures didn't dishearten him and he went on to become one of the greatest pioneers in heart transplantation. In later years, in the 1970s and 1980s, when almost all heart transplantation programmes across the world had been halted, Shumway's unit would be one of only four to continue doing research and transplantations. His focus became rejection and how to beat it.[4]

When he died in 2007, an estimated 60 000 Americans had already received heart transplantations in one of 150 heart-transplantation units in America; 1 240 of these were done at Stanford University.

Adrian Kantrowitz, who had performed the world's second procedure, also did the fifth, shortly after Shumway, this time on an adult. His second patient also didn't survive. Kantrowitz never performed the procedure again, and instead focused on research involving biotechnological interventions to combat heart disease.[5]

He is remembered for his ground-breaking work in developing devices that helped patients with heart trouble. Over a career spanning six decades, he designed and implemented more than 20 medical devices that helped patients with circulation and other vital functions of the heart.[6]

A flood of transplants

The German newspaper *Der Spiegel* asked Barnard why so many hearts were suddenly being transplanted. Was this due to competition between ambitious surgeons? The wait had been so long, but suddenly within six weeks there had been five heart transplants.

Barnard replied, 'I see it differently. I remember as a child we used to go swimming. When the water was cold, everyone stood along the side. No-one wanted to jump in because they didn't know exactly how cold it would be. When one of us eventually jumped in and said it's not that cold, all the rest jumped in too. I believe this was the case with heart transplantation. Many clinics around the world were ready to do it but they were all waiting on one another.'

After the first five heart transplants, the floodgates really opened and surgeons across the world jumped into the fast-moving stream. Although 1968 became the year of the heart, it sadly delivered dismal results. Surgeons everywhere, encouraged by the worldwide media frenzy, performed transplants, often failing miserably.

Most of the surgeons were much less qualified and had much less transplantation experience than Barnard or the Americans. The results were mostly catastrophic, with very few patients surviving.[7]

Barnard also started receiving lashes of criticism, especially from British and American medical circles. The critics said that Barnard had stolen Shumway and Lower's glory by using their research when he performed the first transplant. The irony is that another American, Kantrowitz, had also done a heart transplantation before the more recognised Shumway and Lower. In addition, the work Shumway and Lower had done had been published earlier.

'Some say Chris Barnard stole others' work. The reality is that nothing in medicine stands alone. Naturally, he was aware of the research being done elsewhere. Only an irresponsible fool wouldn't have known. The difference was he had the balls to do what many others already knew was possible,' writes Prof Johan Naudé, an ex-colleague of Barnard's.[8]

In addition, it is undeniable that when it came to results, Barnard and Groote Schuur were outperforming everyone else, including all the Americans. Nevertheless, the controversy followed Barnard for the rest of his life.

Three women and a Pope

After the Blaiberg transplant, Christiaan Barnard went back to Europe without Louwtjie but with Dr MC Botha in tow. They first went to Germany.

Louwtjie later described this visit to Europe as being disastrous for the Barnard family.

Despite all the media coverage and interest, only one South African journalist was sent along on the trip. Peet Simonis had been a journalist for *Volksblad* and later Perskor. He was covering the Christiaan Barnard story for the Sunday newspaper *Dagbreek*.

'In those years, it was mainly sports-desk journalists who got to travel overseas when the Springbok rugby team went on tour.'

Simonis recalls the Barnard trip as being a tremendous story.

'It was a story filled with excitement, enamoured women in Italy, who brought their children so Barnard could touch them, flowers and clothes strewn in the road before him wherever he walked. It was an adulation you cannot imagine.'

It would, however, be the heart surgeon's night-time activities that would get the most media attention, not that Barnard was not warned.

On the flight to Europe, Simonis slipped into the first-class cabin to snap a photo of Barnard.

'When I was leaving, the professor winked at me and said, "You must close your eyes when it comes to the women and things … you know how it goes …" and then he gave a little laugh.'

Simonis replied, 'Professor, you are so well known now, everything you do is newsworthy. If you want to do things you don't want the press to find out about, you'd better be very good at doing it secretly and ensure neither I nor any of the other journalists discover you … And have you heard of the paparazzi in Europe?'

It seems as though Chris did not take the warning seriously.

Travelling on the crest of the Barnard fame, Simonis and Botha didn't even go through customs or immigration.

'German officials moved us past the airport building towards vehicles that were waiting to take us to the Hotel Europa.'

This was where the journalist's path separated from Barnard's for the first time.

In Germany, Chris did a circuit of television and other media interviews. One Friday evening, after a rather disappointing interview, Barnard's host took him out to a nightclub.

Chris wrote about it later: 'The producer came to our table with some female company. One of the women made my heart stop. She had a magnificent body, brown hair, a Slavic appearance with high cheekbones and dark eyes.[9]

'"This is Uta Levka, and this is Prof Barnard,"' the producer introduced us.

"Do you want to dance?" she asked me'.

The two started to dance. Chris was 'hypnotised by the closeness of her body' and didn't notice the camera flashes going off around them.

'We danced away most of the night while we laughed together like old lovers.'

Later, when Barnard signed the guest book, he wrote about an 'unforgettable evening in the arms of one of the most beautiful women in the world'.

The next morning, the newspapers had the photographs and the story on the front pages. Levka turned out to be a famous German actress who was known for her naked scenes in films.[10]

'The reports joked that she usually wore less clothes than my patients did on the operating table.'

Simonis had to deliver an article to *Dagbreek* and was becoming increasingly concerned as time went by in Germany and he had no idea where the professor was. He finally tracked Barnard to Baden-Baden, playground of Germany's rich and famous, and checked into the same hotel, desperate to get his article.

'Shortly before 6.00am that Saturday morning I called Chris's room. To my relief, he answered.

"Heavens Prof, where have you been?"

"The TV people kept me busy all week. But there's trouble – have you seen the newspapers this morning?"

"No? What's going on?"

"Go look in the paper!"

Simonis ran down to the hotel's reception and found the German newspapers filled with photographs of Barnard and Levka.

'There was a photo where Chris is dancing with a pretty woman, his left hand under her jacket. The report states she is Uta Levka (24 years old) and, reading between the lines, it becomes apparent she is no Sunday-school teacher. In addition, there is a juicy bit about how complimentary Chris was to her in the guest book.'

Simonis was still reading the article when Barnard called him back.

'You must try to keep the story out of the South African papers. If my wife sees it, she'll divorce me ...'

'Prof, there's no way the story won't be out in South Africa. I can guarantee you the news wires have distributed it there already. All I can do is to tell your side of the story. So, what is your side of the story?'

Barnard thought a moment before answering:

'What was I supposed to do? I'm a guest of these people and they took me to that place ...'

Chris wrote about what followed in one of his later books. He explains how he was with Uta again on the Saturday evening at a private party but that the two of them never had a moment alone because the paparazzi were everywhere. So they arranged to meet the following day in Munich at a ball that was to be thrown in Barnard's honour at the Hotel Bayerische Hof.

On the dance floor that evening in Munich, the German actress surprised Barnard just as he thought she wasn't going to show after all. Again, they danced the night away. Before she left, Uta handed Chris a note which he read in his room. It contained an address and read 'I hope I will see you later ...'

Chris immediately rushed off to the address.

'Uta was wearing only a very seductive gown. There was no doubt as to the reason why she had invited me to her flat.'[11]

The next step was Rome.

By now the media storm had hit South Africa and another group, Nasionale Pers, sent Louis Louw, a journalist from *Die Burger*, to Italy to cover the rest of the Barnard tour. Louw and Simonis teamed up to cover the remaining part of the tour.

The two introduced themselves as *dottori* (doctors), because people with university degrees may call themselves 'dottori' in Italy. The title certainly opened many doors for the two journalists because, of course, Barnard was a 'dottore' too.

First on Barnard's itinerary was a visit to the Pope, whom he was set to meet in his private office at the Vatican. By this time, Chris had been living out of a suitcase for a while, so his clothes were starting to look creased. He had arrived in Rome on a Sunday and the shops were closed.

'As if in answer to a prayer, the hotel-room phone started ringing. A voice in broken English stated he was here at the hotel to come and take my measurements for my suit in which I was to meet *il Papa*. I invited him up and soon after Angelo Litrico walked into my room.'

The Roman tailor

'"I'm Litrico," he announced himself and stretched to his full height. He must have realised from my reaction that I had no idea who he was, so he continued, "I am Angelo Litrico, tailor of Rome."'

Chris later learnt that Litrico was one of the most famous tailors in the world. He had made suits for world leaders, including US president John F Kennedy and, on the other side of the Iron Curtain, Russian leader Nikita Khruschev. In fact, the shoe that Khruschev had slammed on the table at the United Nations in 1960 in a fit of anger was made by Litrico.

Now Litrico looked at the suit Barnard was wearing and looked horrified.

'Professore, thisa … ees not goot soot for il Papa. You cannot have audience with il Papa dressed in thisa soot.'

'It's a new suit,' Chris said.

'Professore,' he said, his voice dripping with sarcasm, 'that issa all it ees.'

Litrico pulled Barnard's jacket off his back, threw it on the floor and walked all over it to demonstrate his disgust. Barnard was a bit shocked.

'There was nothing wrong with my suit. I had bought it off the shelf in Adderley Street in Cape Town only a week before. I had, in fact, felt completely comfortable in it. It had been a special purchase, intended for my visit with the Pope. In Cape Town, they assured me I was wearing the best.'

Angelo was accompanied by two assistants, one carrying a briefcase and another carrying a huge book of patterns.

'Litrico also discarded my tie and my shirt, asking sarcastically if I had also bought these in Adderley Street. They were clearly all a no for an audience with the Pope.

'The tailor of Rome started measuring me up before I could say anything further. He rattled off commands and comments to his assistants, making it clear that he couldn't believe the professor would dare to walk around in such clothes. He assured me – he, Angelo Litrico – would work till sunrise to ensure I was properly dressed for my visit with *il Papa*. True to his word, Litrico was back by sunrise with a whole new wardrobe. Including new shoes.'

Barnard and Litrico became close friends for many years, until Litrico's untimely death at the age of 58 in 1986.

On Monday morning, 29 January 1968, Barnard first met with the Italian President, after which he had his audience in the Vatican with Pope Paul VI.

'The Pope's personal quarters are in one part of the palace at the Vatican. We ascended the Scala Regia steps, designed by Bernini, and entered a waiting room covered in incredible carpets.'[12]

Chris was accompanied by an Italian doctor who served as a

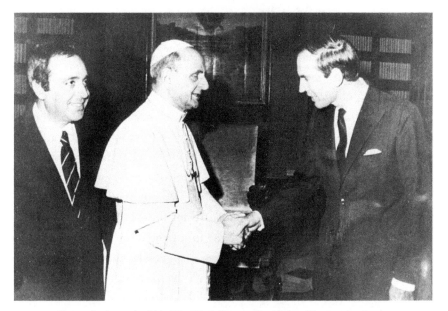

*Towards the end of his life, Chris Barnard said that his meeting in the
Vatican with Pope Paul VI had made the greatest impression on him out of
all his meetings with famous people.*

PHOTOGRAPH COURTESY OF THE HEART OF CAPE TOWN MUSEUM

translator during his meeting with the Pope. They met in his private
office for 20 minutes during which the Pope congratulated him on his
achievement.

The Pope was remarkably well informed when it came to heart transplants and asked many questions that impressed Chris. The audience ran
over its scheduled time due to the Pope's interest in medicine. Barnard
also spoke to the Pope about his own personal struggles relating to faith.[13]

When they finally parted, the Pope told Barnard he would pray for him
and for continued success in his work.

Towards the end of his career, Barnard would highlight his meeting
with the Pope as the most special of his career. Of all the other famous
and interesting people Barnard met, the Pope outshone them all.

Gina and Sophia

The evening after meeting the pope, Barnard attended a party hosted by a famous television producer, where he was introduced to an Italian film star Gina Lollobrigida.

'Gina was wearing hardly any make-up; with her flawless good looks, she hardly needed any. After a few requests, we posed together for some photographs. She was really quite beautiful. For a boy from the Karoo, it was an incredible experience to be so close to such a beautiful actress.'

The two left the party and went dancing in a nightclub together. Later that evening Chris returned to his hotel room alone but with the promise of another meeting at Gina's home the following day.

The next evening Gina was hosting a party at her home and the exhausted Barnard, who was tired from all the partying, fell asleep in her bedroom while she hosted her friends.

Late that night he woke up.

'She was in the room with champagne and two glasses. We celebrated several times that night and I left early the next morning. She took me back to my hotel in her Jaguar. Besides a fur coat, she wasn't wearing anything else. I always wondered what would have happened if we had been in a car accident.'

Lollobrigida fell in love with the South African surgeon and went on to write him passionate love letters, some of which got him into real trouble.

The following afternoon there was a meeting scheduled with another Italian superstar, Sophia Loren. She had suffered a second miscarriage, which had had a huge emotional impact on her. By the end of 1967, Loren was worried that she might never have a baby and she was warned that any further pregnancies could be life threatening. The meeting between her, her husband Carlo Ponti and the miracle doctor from Cape Town in January 1968 was possibly more than simply a social occasion. The meeting may have helped to calm her fears about pregnancy. But this is merely a theory.

Barnard was certainly impressed.

'I admired her greatly. She is everything I admire in a woman: beautiful, highly intelligent, sharp and with a wonderful sense of humour.'

What they discussed remains between them. But in December 1968, after some care from a specialist in Geneva, Loren gave birth to her first son, Carlo Jnr.

The South African journalists also managed to meet the Pontis by using their old trick of referring to themselves as *dottori*. The guards at the Ponti estate let them in believing that they were part of Barnard's team.

'When we arrived at the luxury villa, it was as we had expected – military police, motorbikes, dogs, machine guns, and wet and miserable paparazzi outside the gates where all had been refused entry. We didn't even get out of our car. When a soldier looked in our window we said with puffed-out chests, it was *dottore* Simonis and *dottore* Louw – we are part of Chris Barnard's team. A few words over the radio and the gates swung open, to our great amazement. We were allowed to enter. Close to the front door there was a large living room and there they all were. Chris, Carlo Ponti and, of course, Sophia in all her glory. She was even more beautiful in person than in all her movies. Her sister, who almost matched her in looks, was there too. I've never forgotten the kiss she gave me when we left,' Simonis says.

The highlight of the visit was a tour of Carlo Ponti's personal art collection.

'Louis and I didn't say much. This wasn't a press interview. We were simply "co-doctors" of Prof Chris.'

After Rome, the tour went to London and France. The European tour lasted 10 days in total, and when Barnard returned to South Africa there was a huge media reception at Jan Smuts International Airport in Johannesburg. The stories in the media deriving from the tour had raised the Chris Barnard hysteria a few degrees.

'Chris had to answer many questions arising from his trip to Europe. He did so with aplomb. After all, he hadn't just been having a party. He had appeared before many highly intellectual gatherings and conferences of doctors and specialists and medical institutions. For example, he had been a guest at the famous Max Planck Institute, which was Europe's top medical research institute at the time. Millions of people from around the world started looking at South Africa with new eyes, thanks to Barnard's spontaneous and extraordinary ambassadorial role,' Simonis recalls.

No matter how well Chris could explain away his activities in Europe, there was one person who struggled to accept his actions.

When he arrived back in Cape Town, Louwtjie was not waiting for her husband in the arrivals hall at the airport. She waited outside in the car.

CHAPTER 12

Year of the heart

In CAPE TOWN, BARNARD FOUND PHILIP BLAIBERG WELL ON HIS WAY to recovery. Blaiberg had become a great example of the potential of heart transplantation.

On 2 February 1968, Frederick Prins, the man who had ploughed into Denise Darvall and her mother, was sentenced to two years in jail.[1]

There was bad news relating to the young boy Jonathan, who had received Denise's kidney. The kidney had been successfully transplanted but after some weeks had failed to work and had to be removed. The boy was placed back on dialysis.[2]

Chris spent only a few weeks at home before he left again, this time travelling first to Portugal and then to America, where his first appearance was on Walter Cronkite's television programme, 'Face the Nation'. In the interview, Barnard described himself as 'just a regular guy from a small town in South Africa who had suddenly, overnight, become an expert in everything from ginger biscuits to atomic energy'.[3]

This tour to the United States led to two great controversies. The first was highly personal. It started in Portugal, where Chris had received a bouquet of flowers from Gina Lollobrigida and an accompanying steamy love letter leaving little to the imagination. Chris put the letter in his briefcase. It was a ticking time-bomb.

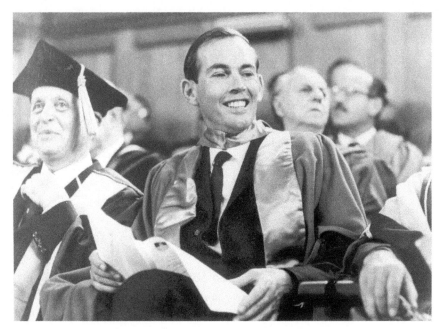

*The University of Cape Town had never before bestowed an honorary degree
on a member of its staff and it had been the policy for many years not to do so.
Until Chris Barnard. Here he is at the ceremony.*

PHOTOGRAPH COURTESY OF THE HEART OF CAPE TOWN MUSEUM

March 1968, San Francisco

Louwtjie joined Chris in America, despite – or perhaps because of – the
scandals arising from the European trip in January. Chris had managed
to convince Louwtjie that the scandals had largely been the result of
media speculation, without much substance. She had believed him to
some extent.

The trip started out well, but the wheels came off in San Francisco.

Barnard had been invited to do a presentation to the members of the
American College of Cardiology in the Hilton Hotel in San Francisco.
He was to present on the outcomes of his two heart transplants to a
room filled with around 3 000 top cardiologists and other specialists,
including many of his greatest competitors and critics.[4]

It was the first time so many of the world's top surgeons had gathered together in one venue and the occasion was to listen to what Barnard had to say. It was truly a huge moment for the professor from Cape Town, to get the acknowledgement of his peers, people who truly understood what it had meant to do Washkansky's heart transplant.

For this big occasion, Barnard had prepared a set of slides that he would show to the audience while delivering his address.

Louwtjie had decided to stay behind in the hotel room while Chris was preparing for his presentation in the ballroom. Shortly before he was due to start, Chris realised that two of his slides were missing. He called the hotel room from the lobby and asked his wife to look for the slides in his briefcase.

Louwtjie recalls what happened next: 'Chris asked me to look in his briefcase, where I came upon the love letters written by an international film star [Lollobrigida] – evidence of his love affairs in Europe that he had denied. I was shocked, lost and alone and fell into a pit of despair. I walked over to the window and decided suicide would be the quickest way to get out of this.'[5]

This was a bitter pill for Louwtjie to swallow after Chris had promised her that the rumours and stories about him and 'La Lollo' were only media speculation.

Down in the ballroom, Chris got worried when Louwtjie didn't appear, so he stormed up to the 23rd-floor bedroom. There he found his wife at the open window.

It seemed as if she was about to jump.

Chris recalls that he made a decision to leave Louwtjie there.

'My presence wouldn't change anything. It would be best to leave her alone and pray that she changed her mind,' Barnard recalls in *Tweede Lewe*.

He left the room and went back downstairs without the slides.

In the ballroom, Chris found his audience ready and waiting, and he went to stand in front of them.

He waited, listening for the sirens. Nothing! Would she go through with it?

159

Loud applause pulled him back to reality. He had to speak.

Initially he appeared to be terribly nervous. But then he broke the ice by telling a joke about a chauffeur who swopped places with a well-known heart surgeon one day during a publicity tour. The chauffeur, who had heard the talk many times before, managed to pull off a great show but at question time he was asked a tough question by a renowned surgeon who happened to be in the audience. The quick-thinking chauffeur said that the question was so easy that he'd leave the answer to the chauffeur in the back of the hall.

The joke worked and the ice was broken. The rest of Barnard's talk went brilliantly and he delivered an excellent lecture on heart transplantation to the packed hall, illustrated with his slides.

At the end of the talk there was a standing ovation. Barnard was acknowledged by the people who understood best what his accomplishment meant.

He made another big mistake that day.

He didn't give much credit to the other pioneers in heart transplantation – many of whom had done much of the research on which his work had been based and were in the room. Richard Lower was one of the real pioneers who were present that day.[6]

'All the early pioneers of cardiology and heart transplantation were in the audience. All Chris should have done was show a little humility and said, "We have done this and that, but we were really building on the work all of you had done". Except he never referred to anyone besides himself. It was just me, me, me. After the lecture, I saw him by himself and went to greet him,' Lower recalled later.

What the surgeons, including Lower, didn't know about was the situation in the hotel room on the 23rd floor.

After Chris had left, Louwtjie decided to turn away from the window.

'I had stood at the open window, high above the street. Far below I could see the people and cars moving around like ants. A single step would have been enough to end it all. Then it would all have been quiet. I felt a soft hand on my shoulder and turned around, but there was nobody there. The bright faces of my children in a photo on the bedside table caught my eye. They saved me. I couldn't do them any harm. I smoked a cigarette and fell asleep on the bed,' Louwtjie recalled in her memoir.

And that was where Chris found her.

A portion of the contents of one of Lollobrigida's love letters was later published in Louwtjie's memoir and then distributed further in the tabloids.

Lollobrigida promptly sued Chris and Louwtjie Barnard. The Italian actress claimed that publishing the contents of her letter was an invasion of her privacy. She acknowledged that she had been in love with Barnard, but that it was over.

'I couldn't blame myself for having genuine feelings for a man the entire world had fallen in love with.'[7]

Despite the enormous personal crisis, the Barnards continued with their tour and their lives, living like two strangers.

From San Francisco, they went to Minnesota, where they stayed with the Wangensteens. While they were there, the next big crisis in heart transplantation erupted.

An American senator from Minnesota, Walter Mondale, wanted to bring in legislation to create a commission that would oversee medical research.[8] He was worried about the ethical, legal and social implications pertaining to the highly technical and advanced new medical practices, that were taking the world by storm. He highlighted heart transplantation and genetic manipulation as areas of scientific advancement that were raising serious questions.[9]

Between 8 March 1968 and 2 April 1968, the Senate Committee on Government Operations held senate hearings into the matter.[10] The implications were serious for the medical fraternity in the United States. Both Barnard and Wangensteen were requested to appear in Washington DC to provide evidence at the hearings.

The Mondale hearings of 1968

Barnard and his erstwhile mentor, Wangensteen, appeared before one of the hearings.[11]

Barnard later wrote that he felt the committee was political and aimed at garnering political publicity. As an outsider, he didn't pull his punches. He was not beholden to anyone at the hearings and not dependent on American legislators and American funding for his work.

Chris came out firing on behalf of his medical colleagues and delivered some key testimony.

'[The chairperson] asked me if I thought the average man on the street should have a say in heart transplantation, how they get done and which donors should be used. When I said no, the doctor is the expert and these matters should be in the doctor's hands, he asked me who pays for the operations in South Africa. I replied the provincial government. He looked quite pleased with himself and said – so, the taxpayer? I said yes. Then he said since taxpayers pay for the operation, surely they have a right to have a say in the matter?'

Chris said no and asked the chairperson who was paying for the Vietnam War. Wasn't it the American taxpayer? The chairman agreed.

'Then I said, since the taxpayers were paying for the war, surely they have a right to tell the generals when to attack and which weapons to use?'[12]

The press gallery laughed out loud.[13]

Barnard, who was already known for thinking on his feet, embarrassed Mondale with further comments about the potential implications of an oversight committee. He warned the senator that the proposed oversight commission would threaten American medical research and would be an insult for American doctors.

'If I was in competition with my colleagues in this country – which I am not – then I would welcome this commission because it would put the [American] doctors so far behind and would restrict them so much they would never be able to catch up,' Barnard stated.[14]

A large number of other scientists and specialists provided testimony at the hearings, largely in opposition to Mondale's plan.[15]

Kantrowitz argued that doctors were entering areas in the development of medicine where a certain amount of courage was needed for success.

'I'm not sure that committees have a reputation for boldness and courage.'

Mondale's efforts resulted in a much-weakened version of a commission, which was eventually established in 1974.[16]

In later years, Mondale became the 42nd American Vice-President to Jimmy Carter. In 1984, he was the unsuccessful Democratic presidential candidate, losing to Ronald Reagan.

On 25 May 1968, Richard Lower performed his first human-to-human heart transplant in Virginia. It was the world's 16th procedure. The patient was Joseph Kleet, who died a week later. This operation was to cause enormous legal problems for Lower and nearly led to his imprisonment.

Following Kleet's death, a lawsuit was brought against Lower by the family of the donor. Lower was charged with murder and the family wanted to sue him for US$1 million. The case would come down to the question of when organ donors may be declared dead. The case dragged on for four years, during which time Lower was not allowed to perform any more transplants. Lower was finally vindicated when the judge declared that brain death in patients could be accepted as the norm to determine when a person is dead.

The Cape Town symposium

Chris Barnard arranged an International Symposium with the world's top cardiologists and heart surgeons in Cape Town on 12 July 1968. He invited the leaders from all 15 medical centres that had performed heart transplants at that stage. The provincial government covered the costs for the event. All the invited delegates, except Shumway and Lower, accepted the invitation. Among the attendees were Kantrowitz and Cooley.[17]

Some of the American and British media were still quite critical of Barnard and claimed his success was due to luck because he happened to have a donor and a patient at the right time.

In reality, the media was struggling to explain how an unknown team of South African surgeons with much less funding and fewer resources had managed to achieve what the Americans and European surgeons had been unable to do.

The American and British media also forgot to mention how well Groote Schuur's heart-transplant patients were doing compared to those with the best American doctors, including Shumway.

The first three heart-transplant patients of Shumway's Stanford team survived for 15, 3 and 46 days, respectively. The first three patients operated on by the Groote Schuur team under Barnard survived for 18, 593 and 621 days, respectively.

The symposium was a great success, despite the absence of Shumway and Lower.

Kantrowitz commented at the time, 'Christiaan Barnard is doing it better than all of us and that's why we're here.'[18]

Blaiberg goes home

Philip Blaiberg was released from hospital 74 days after his heart transplant, on 21 July 1968.

There were thousands of people waiting outside the hospital to see Blaiberg. The world's third heart-transplant patient was in a wheelchair inside the hospital but stood up close to the doors, saying he would walk out under his own steam.

The nursing staff watched from the balconies above the exit as Blaiberg shook Barnard's hand before getting into a chauffeur-driven car to be whisked away to his home in Wynberg.

'For the man who was ready to say goodbye to the world, the world's reply is a great hello,' says the voice-over on the old black-and-white television footage reflecting the event on YouTube.

The first half of the year had flown by like a dream. Chris and Louwtjie's relationship was still tense but the couple went on three further trips overseas, to Spain, Iran and England. In Tehran, Barnard received a gift of some valuable Persian carpets.

This turned out to be the last trip the married couple would ever go on together. Louwtjie and Chris had a fight on the night of a big celebratory gala dinner and Louwtjie refused to attend it. For her, the crowds and attention following her husband around were getting to be too much. She felt as if she were the prey surrounded by human vultures.

'I felt like a dead person among all the living.'

There was little fighting spirit left in Louwtjie.

'By this time there were so many women in his life that I had to either take no notice of them or I had to accept them.'

Louwtjie returned to South Africa and Chris went on to London where, in the space of a single day, he found comfort in the arms of three different women, one of whom was the famous French singer Françoise Hardy. Hardy was performing in the Savoy Hotel where Chris was staying.[19]

Princess Grace

The final nail in the coffin of the Barnard marriage was the famous Red Cross Ball in Monaco. Chris was invited to attend as an honoured guest by Prince Rainier and his wife, Princess Grace. The ball was to be held in August.

'I asked him to take me with to the ball and asked if he'd buy me a pretty dress for the occasion. He said I wasn't invited and couldn't go. It was like a death sentence,' Louwtjie wrote.

At this time Marius Barnard was increasingly taking charge of the heart transplant team in the absence of his brother. Marius also recalled that the Red Cross Ball had caused huge conflict between his brother and Louwtjie.

'She pleaded with him not to attend.'

Chris insisted on going.

'I'm determined to attend the Red Cross Ball, even if Louwtjie says that if I go our marriage is over. Which person working for a government salary and who gets invited by royalty to be an honoured guest, refuses the invitation?'

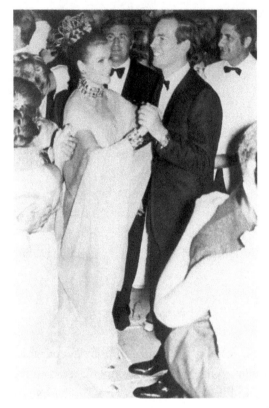

*The Red Cross Ball in Monaco was a great occasion and Chris
Barnard was an honoured guest, seated beside princess Grace. It
caused a great rift in his first marriage but Barnard insisted on going.*

PHOTOGRAPH COURTESY OF THE HEART OF CAPE TOWN MUSEUM

The Monaco Red Cross Ball with Princess Grace was *the* social event
on the European calendar.[20] Litrico made Chris a special dinner jacket
for the occasion.

Chris attended the ball on 10 August 1968. He found himself seated
to the left of Princess Grace and he had the honour of having the second
dance of the evening with her. For Chris, the princess was 'more beautiful than I could have dreamt'.

The photos of the two circulated around the world.

In Cape Town, the media also made a big fuss about the photographs of Chris and Princess Grace.

During his visit to Monaco, Chris also met the son of the ex-Italian dictator, Benito Mussolini. The young man was a well-known pianist.

'I couldn't help thinking how quickly things can change,' Chris wrote later.

Louwtjie had finally had enough and she threw Chris's clothes out in black plastic bags. In addition, in a fit of anger and sadness, she threw the expensive Persian carpets they had received in Iran out in the rain, with the rubbish.

Dorothy Fischer

Groote Schuur's third heart transplant was performed on 7 September 1968 on Pieter Smith, a 52-year-old policeman. He received the heart of a 38-year-old domestic servant named Evelyn Jacobs, who had suffered a massive brain haemorrhage and had been unconscious since she was admitted to Groote Schuur.

Initially her name was withheld in line with a new protocol that had been adopted following the International Heart Symposium in Cape Town. This led to a tremendous furore for some time after the operation. Newspapers mistakenly identified another woman as the donor and splashed the information across their front pages, including exposés of how the woman's family had not been informed about the transplant. Surgeons were even branded as 'organ vultures'.

The authorities then released Jacobs' particulars.

'I initially had no problem with naming the donors, but what is happening is that newspapers are digging up everything they can about the families of donors and if they find some skeletons they have no hesitation in coming out with the full details,' Barnard explained in an article in the *Cape Times*.

This operation was the 42nd in the world.

In April 1969, the Groote Schuur team made further history when they

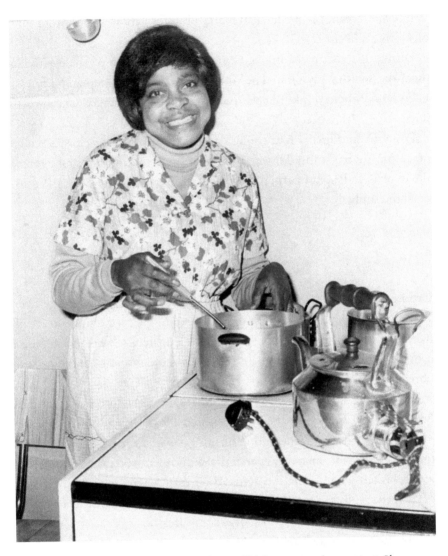

Dorothy Fischer was Groote Schuur's fifth heart-transplant patient. She would survive for 13 years and insisted on calling Barnard 'Papa'.

PHOTOGRAPH COURTESY OF THE HEART OF CAPE TOWN MUSEUM

did two heart transplants. First, on 7 April 1969, Douglas Killops (63 years old) received a new heart; he died 64 days later. This operation was followed by another that became Barnard's greatest triumph – the transplant he performed on 17 April.

Dorothy Fischer was a 38-year-old woman whose heart had been damaged by rheumatic fever when she was a child. Fischer was Chris Barnard's fifth heart transplant patient and the first woman to receive a heart transplant. At the time of her operation, Dorothy was dying and the expectation was that she had, at best, nine weeks left.

The transplant was a great success.

For the rest of her life, Fischer called Barnard 'Papa'.[21] 'Because Papa gave me a new heart.'

Dorothy went on to live another 13 years with her new heart.

In an interview given nine years after her heart transplant, Dorothy said it had all been worth it. 'It meant a new life.'

Marius Barnard commented that in Fischer's case, no-one could argue against the fact that hers was a perfect result.

Marius said the Groote Schuur team would continue to do heart transplantations where needed.

'It's an acceptable treatment for people with a cardiological condition that cannot be helped in any other way. It is a necessity today and should be done in instances where it could provide someone with a longer life. It's no different than removing a burst appendix.'[22]

Heart-transplant moratoriums

Around the world the mad rush to perform heart transplants started to die down following the large amounts of negative press relating to the mostly negative results from accross the globe. Most patients were still dying – and within days of the operation, if not on the table itself.

By April 1969, 133 hearts transplants had been done across the world; only 13 patients were still alive.

There were, however, some successes and further progress. Denton

Cooley in Texas had done 5 000 open-heart operations by this time, as well as 17 heart transplants. On 4 April 1969, Cooley used an artificial heart for the first time in a patient, managing to keep the patient alive for 63 hours when no donor heart was available.[23]

The media attention had placed huge pressure on surgeons across the globe who had too often attempted the procedure with unprepared teams. The ensuing bad outcomes caused much reputational damage to heart transplantation. However, even the best American surgeons were still struggling to keep their patients alive. Again, the exception was Groote Schuur. Patients who received heart transplants in Cape Town outperformed the global statistics on every level. Blaiberg was still alive and had even written a book about his experiences, in which he described how it felt to hold his own heart in his hands. Sadly, however, even the Cape Town team didn't have all the answers yet and Blaiberg's time was also running out.

By this time, Louwtjie had decided to leave Chris and, on 23 May 1969, she filed for a divorce in the Cape Town High Court. Their divorce was finalised two months later.[24]

Blaiberg dies

The Cape Town dentist, Philip Blaiberg, survived another 19 months and 15 days with his second heart. In the process, he became a symbol of hope across the world at a time when most heart-transplant patients were dying of infection or rejection or other complications within days of the procedure.

On 17 August 1969, Blaiberg died of chronic rejection. His body's cells had gradually been destroying the cells in his new heart until it could no longer function.

Eileen Blaiberg had always known that there was no guarantee her Phil would keep on living.

'What we received was a gift to us, a time during which we were so happy. I shall never forget the look on Phil's face when he left the hospital after receiving his new heart. He was unaware of the media and the police and the crowds of people who were all there to see him. He just stood there and took a deep breath and said, "Fresh air. Beautiful fresh air."

'[At the end] I was allowed in the room to be at his side. I knew I was saying goodbye to my husband. Our wonderful, short bonus period was over. That evening, Dr Barnard called me and said my husband was dying. He said he wanted to ask one question – was it all worth it? I answered it was every bit worth it.'

Eileen described how she and Philip had rediscovered everything together.

'It was as if I was also seeing everything again for the first time. We discovered a new world. Together we saw the world was a wonderful place. Slowly we picked up our lives again. The doctors were always close but at least Phil was at home. When visitors would ask if he needed anything, he'd say why – do I look sick? He wasn't interested in material things any more and always kept saying everything will be okay. He was so optimistic.

'How many people get a second chance at life? Phil lived another 594 days and we enjoyed most of them. Prof Barnard said he would be continuing with heart transplants and said only patients could say at the end of it, if it was worth it. Phil said yes. I also say yes. I was grateful for every minute of every extra day that Phil received. I have so many happy memories I would not have had otherwise.'[25]

Philip Blaiberg's death renewed the public's scepticism about heart transplantation although surgeons still believed in the procedure. DeBakey said transplants were justified if they could prolong a patient's life, even for a year or two.

Kantrowitz said Blaiberg's case was a tremendous accomplishment – even greater than man landing on the moon. 'The task of saving the lives of hundreds of thousands of critically ill patients is at least as important as discovering the Universe.'[26]

The months that Blaiberg had lived with his transplanted heart was the realisation of a dream that was shared by the world's heart surgeons.

Status of organ transplantation at 18 August 1969

Heart transplants: 142 operations, 32 survivors

Lung transplants: 20 operations, 10 survivors

Pancreas transplants: 10 operations, 10 survivors

Liver transplants: 100 operations, 14 survivors

Kidney transplants: 2 321 operations.

(First-year survival rate of kidney transplant patients with family donors: 87%. First-year survival rate with non-family donors: 42%)[27]

CHAPTER 13

Love in the days of medicine

O N THE HOME FRONT, LOVE WAS IN THE AIR.
Barbara Zoellner was a beautiful Johannesburg socialite. She was the teenage daughter of a wealthy mining magnate, Fred Zoellner, and his wife Ursula (Ulli). The relationship between Barbara and the heart surgeon had the blessing of Barbara's parents. Barnard was a catch, after all.

The French magazine *Paris Match* had rated Barnard as one of the four most desirable lovers in the world. The other three on the list were Princess Astrid from Belgium, the tennis player Bjorn Borg and Greek heiress Christina Onassis.

Once his divorce from Louwtjie was finalised, the relationship with Barbara picked up speed, and six months after the divorce, on 14 February 1970, the 47-year-old Chris Barnard got married for the second time. His new bride was 19 years old.

The marriage ceremony was held shortly after midnight at the home of Barbara's parents in Johannesburg and was attended by only a few close friends and family, who served as witnesses when the magistrate made things official.[1]

Barbara didn't want to get married on Friday the 13th, due to the superstition attached to the date, so the couple had waited to just after midnight.[2]

Less than half an hour after the ceremony, Barnard threw open the gates to the estate and offered all the assembled journalists glasses of

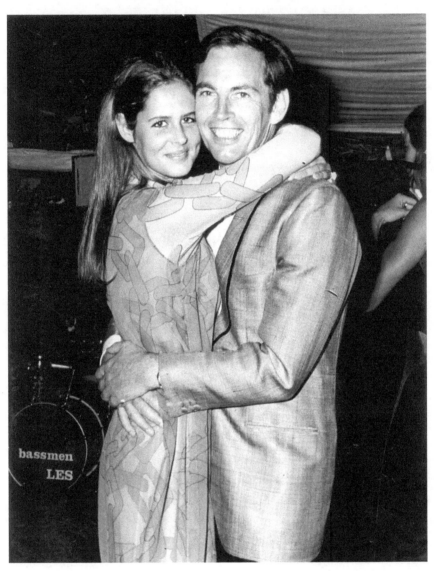

*In 1970 Chris Barnard married 19-year-old Barbara Zoellner. This
photo was taken at their engagement party.*

champagne. He apologised for having made them stand outside.[3]

'It's not because I don't like you. It's important, however, to have a certain amount of privacy in one's life,' Barnard said as he handed out the alcohol.[4]

He denied rumours that he and Barbara were emigrating. The rumours had resulted from his continued criticism of the South African government's racist segregation policies. Barnard said that he would be returning after his honeymoon and the couple would be settling in Cape Town.[5] They would spend a few days in Italy before going to the United States.

Three days later, on 17 February, a photograph in the *Chicago Tribune* showed the happy couple on honeymoon in Italy, pictured on the balcony of their hotel room. The couple had a difficult time in Italy due to the media and public frenzy that went with them. Earlier they had been forced to cancel all sightseeing trips for fear of being harassed by Rome's notoriously aggressive paparazzi. In an earlier run-in with the paparazzi, the new Mrs Barnard's stockings were torn to shreds and her shoes were ripped off.[6]

No more hearts

On 10 May 1971, Chris Barnard performed his first heart transplant in two years. The patient was a policeman, Dirk van Zyl (44 years old). The donor was Damon Meyer (24 years old), a farmworker who had fallen out of a tree.

Van Zyl was Barnard's sixth heart transplant and became Groote Schuur's greatest success story, eventually living for 23 years with his new heart. Van Zyl's recovery was so good that he returned to work three months after his transplant and never missed a single day of work until his retirement, 15 years later.[7]

By this time, Chris had become tremendously frustrated by doctors who were no longer referring patients to him.

'Doctors at Groote Schuur don't share my view that heart transplants are an acceptable medical treatment.'[8]

Marius Barnard later wrote in his memoir about the attitude of some of their colleagues towards the heart-transplant unit.

'The Department of Neurology was our main source of suitable donors since they worked with fatal head injuries that often led to patients being declared brain dead. The Department of Neurology, however, was never very keen to help us – in fact, some of them were aggressively obstructive. I even complained about it in writing to the head of the department, but nothing changed.'

Possibly, the larger medical fraternity at Groote Schuur were buying into the worldwide concerns about heart transplantation, rather than focusing on the incredible results their own unit was achieving.

Some months earlier, on 25 February 1971, Marius had performed a heart transplant. The Barnards were the first set of brothers to perform the intricate procedure.

The next big thing

Chris Barnard's next big breakthrough was achieved on 25 July 1971. This time, Chris performed a simultaneous heart and double lung transplantation on Adrian Herbert. Herbert had been bedridden for two years with an incurable lung condition that had dramatically weakened his heart.

After the operation, Barnard was severely criticised because they said that his operation on Herbert had ignored the recent setbacks in transplantation.[9]

In typical fighting fashion, Barnard retorted, 'They must judge me on my results, not on their own experiences. I treat my patients because I want to do what is best for them, despite criticism involving my reputation. If this patient had not received this operation, he would not have survived. The operation was his last chance.'

Herbert died 23 days later of pneumonia, but the operation was considered to be a huge accomplishment. Following two similar earlier operations done elsewhere in the world, the patients had not survived beyond two days.[10]

Following the Herbert operation, there was a new controversy and it involved the use of the organs that had belonged to Jackson Gunya, a 28-year-old black man. There was some confusion around the marriage status of Gunya and whether the hospital had received the necessary permission to use his organs. The provincial administration stated that, despite all efforts, no next of kin could be found in time. Permission for use of the organs was then provided as per legislation and involved the provincial pathologist and the Attorney General of the Cape Province.[11]

Barnard simply stated that his transplant team had done everything by the book. As always, the team had no say about donors or organ donation.

It turned out that Gunya was married to a woman named Rosalie and they had two sons. Rosalie was justifiably upset at the time but the provincial head of health, Lapa Munnik, maintained that the hospital had not broken any laws.

The tragic reality of apartheid legislation colours in the rest of the story. Rosalie was living in Cape Town illegally – in contravention of the Group Areas Act – and didn't qualify to live with her husband. Accordingly, when the authorities visited Jackson Gunya's official place of residence, there was no evidence of a wife to be found.

On 14 November 1971, Barnard performed his eighth heart transplant. The 62-year-old Lindsay Rich received the heart of Robert Nixon.[12]

Rich commented ahead of the operation: 'Which person of my age would not cling to the last spark of hope of a normal life?'[13]

Rich died 12 days later.[14]

Both Fischer and Van Zyl were still alive and doing very well.

Across the globe, the handbrake was being pulled up and moratoriums were increasingly being placed on the procedure. Following the rush of transplants in 1968 and 1969, in 1971, only 17 heart transplants were performed globally.[15]

Most hospitals had stopped doing the procedure and this was the case throughout the rest of the 1970s. Only four centres continued to perform heart transplants. These were Stanford (Shumway), the Medical College of Virginia (Lower), Hôpital Universitaire Pitié-Salpêtrière in Paris (Christian Cabrol) and Groote Schuur (Barnard).[16]

Remarkably, three of these surgeons had studied under Lillehei and Wangensteen and the fourth – Lower – had studied under Shumway.[17]

Chris and Barbara

Chris and Barbara were a glamourous couple, travelling the world from great cities to tiny rural towns like Jansenville in the Eastern Cape, where they attended the town's 10th annual agricultural show in March 1972. The two were treated like royalty and Barbara was crowned the Mohair Queen.

Overseas, Barnard remained popular. He was still corresponding with Sophia Loren – mostly pertaining to Italian children with heart conditions. Loren even named a special pasta dish in Barnard's honour – Pasticatta alla Christiaan Barnard.

The moratoriums that had been put in place since the December 1967 breakthrough at Groote Schuur were a great concern for Barnard. On a visit to London in May 1972, Chris described the situation as a 'great tragedy'.

'People are dying today who need not be dying.'[18]

Barnard said that progress was being held back because doctors had stopped exploring the boundaries of cardiac medicine.

'When man started to fly, there were many crashes but that didn't stop man from trying to fly. We've had many crashes in heart surgery but that's no reason to stop doing it. That's the sad part of it, that as soon as we are faced with failure we throw our hands up in the air.'

Barnard blamed the media as well for their role in the situation regarding heart transplantation and said they had frightened off potential patients. He also slammed unprepared doctors who had jumped on the bandwagon and caused great harm because they tackled the complex procedure without the requisite experience and knowledge.

Finally, Barnard also stated that superstition, perpetuated by people who weren't comfortable with the idea of a foreign heart in their bodies, was another problem leading to the lack of progress.

He told the *Guardian* that opposition to him personally in South Africa had also contributed to the fact that fewer and fewer patients were being referred to him.

'It's difficult to understand if one considers the initial results for liver transplantations were even worse than those for hearts, yet liver transplantations are still going on.'

Barnard was getting special leave from his bosses for all his ongoing trips across the globe – leave that had to be authorised months ahead of time by the hospital's management, as well as the provincial cabinet. He was considered to be 'on official duty for the period of his absence'.[19]

Barnard's travel and accommodation costs were covered by the entities that invited him abroad. In America, for example, Barnard's last visit had been paid for by Johnson & Johnson, who accommodated him in a suite in the Park Lane Hotel in New York.

Globally, Barnard was still adored by the public. He went with Barbara to Athens, Greece, for his 50th birthday celebration in November 1972.

On the day of their departure, thousands of Greek heart patients from all across Greece turned out at Athens International Airport, desperate to be examined by the South African heart doctor. According to the *Sunday Times* on 19 November 1972, the airport was turned into a field hospital. 'When Prof Barnard entered the airport concourse, he was visibly moved by the scene awaiting him. "I will only see the children," he said and set up surgery in the Olympic Airways clinic at the airport.'

In the four hours before he was due to fly back to Johannesburg, he saw about 100 children, who went in and out of the clinic 'as if on a conveyor belt'.

Back home, the lack of transplant patients continued to be a huge frustration and, in April 1973, Barnard told *The New York Times* yet again that doctors were no longer referring patients to him.

'In six months, we haven't done one [heart transplant] operation because we had no patients. When we finally get one, the doctors won't tell us if they have potential donors.'

By 1973, Barnard had performed 10 heterotopic heart transplantations. Four patients survived longer than 18 months, one lived for 13 years and another for 23 years. Barnard's record was unsurpassed.[20]

Under Barnard's dictatorial surgical style, Sister Jordaan often rued the day she was born but, nevertheless, always considered it an honour to work with Barnard.[21]

'He had an incredibly high standard for the total healthcare of his patients and expected the same level from doctors, nurses and emergency personnel. I believe these high standards were the reasons why the Groote Schuur heart unit had such excellent results.'

Jordaan said that Barnard's patients were all treated equally well regardless of religious belief, race or nationality.[22]

In 1973, the surgical team at Groote Schuur performed 442 operations; 82 were closed-heart operations and 353 were open-heart procedures. Of the 442 patients, 220 were white. The rest were black, coloured and Indian. All Barnard's patients received the same treatment; they were treated in the same wards with the same equipment and by the same doctors.

Piggyback hearts

On 25 November 1974, Barnard performed his first heart transplant in more than a year. This time he used a new technique, one he would call the *abbahart* or piggyback technique. The new technique consisted of implanting a donor heart into the body of a patient without removing the donor's old, sick heart. The new heart served to assist the patient's old heart. The beauty of this new technique was that it limited rejection and gave patients a greater chance of survival.

The idea was partly inspired by Chris's eldest son, André. A man who had become like a second father to André, Martin Franzot, had been Barnard's ninth heart-transplant patient. Tragically, Franzot died on the operating table on 16 August 1972.[23]

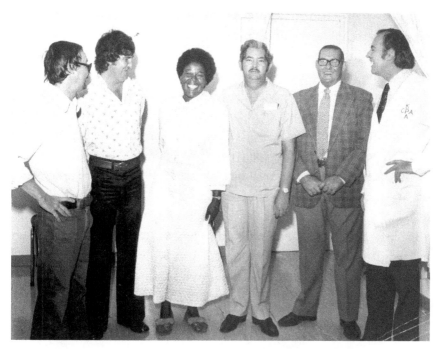

In this photograph taken at one of the anniversary events for the first heart transplant, Barnard is on the far right. Pictured are some of the patients who received piggyback heart transplants.

André was in tears and kept asking his father why he hadn't rather left Franzot's old heart in place. At least then his friend would still be alive. Following this question, Barnard started experimenting with the idea of a piggyback heart.

'The old heart can do what it can, and what it cannot, the new heart can kick in to take up the load. It works like two farm dams: when one is full, it spills over into the other one and relieves the pressure on the first one,' Barnard explained.

In the first piggyback operation, the heart of a 10-year-old girl was attached to the heart of 58-year-old Ivor Taylor in an operation that took five hours. The two hearts worked independently, which meant the patients had two heartbeats.

'The new operation had good results. From 1974, Chris would use the piggyback technique in all his transplants, until his retirement in 1983,' Marius recalled.[24]

Three of the first five piggyback heart patients survived for longer than 10 years. Taylor, however, died four months after his operation.[25]

Where the heterotopic transplantations had a one-year and five-year survival rate of 40% and 20%, respectively, this increased to 60% and 36%, respectively, when the piggyback procedure was introduced.[26]

Groote Schuur Hospital would eventually do 49 piggyback procedures on 43 patients over the next nine years.[27]

Further intensive research work was becoming difficult for Barnard after his heart transplantation work. He was travelling the world and his arthritis was wreaking havoc on his hands. On some days, when the disease flared up, he could hardly button his own shirts.

Still, Barnard kept pushing the surgical boundaries, and on 21 June 1977, in an effort to save an Italian patient's life, he transplanted a baboon heart into her chest using the piggyback technique. The team had initially tried to rebuild her badly damaged heart but when it wouldn't start beating once it was taken off bypass, the decision was made to implant the baboon heart. The woman lived for another five and a half hours.

Barnard said that a human heart would probably have kept her alive. 'But it is a matter of availability. You don't have a donor just when you ask for it.'[28]

Barnard did realise, though, that a baboon heart would not be able to perform the functions of a human heart because it was not big enough. Barnard had stated before the operation that he would consider such an operation only as a last resort in trying to save a patient's life.

In October 1977, Barnard took his last step across the boundaries of medical science when he transplanted a chimpanzee's heart into Benjamin Fortes, a 59-year-old chartered accountant from Cape Town. This was not a success either and it became Chris Barnard's last experiment with animal organs.

Barnard said at the time that animal hearts would probably not be able to provide much beyond temporary help for dying patients.

'The rejection happens too fast. It's almost instantaneous that the human body starts rejecting the foreign tissue.'

Working with children

Barnard's personal life had become more interesting to the scandal-seeking media than his professional work. Sadly, he is hardly remembered for the incredible work he did with children at the Red Cross War Memorial Children's Hospital. Yet, in his later life, he said that it was this work that he considered his true legacy, even more so than the heart transplant.

Dr Otto Thaning was a registrar working under Barnard at the children's hospital.

'He always expected 110% from you. And it was never personal. He simply expected utter professionalism. He demanded it from himself.'

Thaning says that it was under Barnard's leadership that the Red Cross War Memorial Children's Hospital desegregated its intensive-care wards in the early 1970s, despite a backlash from the government, which was still hell bent on implementing its segregationist laws.

'I phoned him one evening and said we were going to put the children from wards C and D (one white, one black) together into one ward. He said that's fine.'

Thaning says there was huge pressure on Barnard to reverse this decision, but he refused to back down.

'Some were worried that white families would be unhappy about the fact that their children were in mixed wards. One morning when we walked into the ward, there was a white father who had taken a huge teddy bear to his child and he saw all the black children from desperately poor areas lying in the other beds. The next morning the father brought teddy bears for all the other children in the ward. I phoned Prof Barnard and told him we were going to be okay.'

Bob Molloy was a journalist with the *Cape Argus* newspaper. He wrote later that the pressure was always increasing on Barnard.

'His every step was watched for every bit of innuendo and there was always a camera lens close to snap him with every woman that came close to him.'[29]

Molloy says that Barnard's career cost him a lot of personal sacrifice.

'In return, he was paid a state wage that never amounted to much more than that of a good hairdresser.'[30]

Don Mackenzie, an old friend of Barnard's, reiterated this.

'Chris knew how to turn a penny. He had to. At the time of the heart transplant, he was earning R500 a month. I was a professional photographer and I was earning around R3 000 per month. Except Chris was the one with five medical degrees and he'd just transplanted a heart.'

Molloy says that when it came to the media, Chris Barnard could never see that it was a one-way street.

'Barnard knocking became a sport. But he was never an easy target. The British media especially had it in for him. There was a long-running vendetta with the TV personality David Frost. Frost had held a few debates on live television with Barnard and had lost. He was humiliated. So Frost sent some agents to South Africa to dig up dirt on Barnard that he would air in Barnard's absence. Chris would always say it was like bowling at the stumps when the batsman wasn't at the crease. One day Frost set an ambush for Barnard in the USA. He caught Chris off guard after a long flight and blamed Chris for all the evils of apartheid on air. Barnard reacted with long-winded explanations of what was happening in South Africa and it came across as a defence of apartheid. He should simply have said he agreed as he was on the same side – which he was. It was the best journalism hatchet job ever. Barnard lasted a long time but at the end even he wasn't able to withstand media manipulation,' Molloy recalled.[31]

Bureaucracy

The human tragedy of a patient awaiting an organ for transplantation is often seen only from the patient's view. For the surgeons, it could be just as traumatic.[32]

In a column in the *Cape Times*, Barnard recounted the feeling of a patient who was dying and knew it.

'He knew his only hope of survival was dependent on the death of someone else. It is one of the more macabre aspects of transplantation surgery, one that has a strong psychological effect on the people on the receiving end of it. The patient knew the chances of getting an organ were small and he accepted it with courage, even towards the end when it became clear, even to him, that he was nearing the end.'

By the end of the 1970s, the bureaucracy had increased the red tape relating to organ donation and this led to huge delays – delays that often meant that by the time all the boxes had been ticked, the organs were no longer feasible.

'Families were still coming to us with hope. Ours [transplantation programme] had been considered to be the best, with the best results, but then we had to start explaining how South Africa, once considered to be the world leader in transplantation, had now hedged the donation of organs with legislation. Legislation that made the possibility of getting healthy donor hearts more a miracle than a possibility. While lots of other, valuable cardiac surgery was happening, especially on children, the era of South African heart transplantation was basically over.'[33]

Barnard compared the bitterness of losing to sucking on an old copper coin.

'If you ever want to know what real loss or failure feels like, try spending a hard night at work trying to save a patient's life and then go home the next morning as the sun is rising, knowing it was all for nothing.'[34]

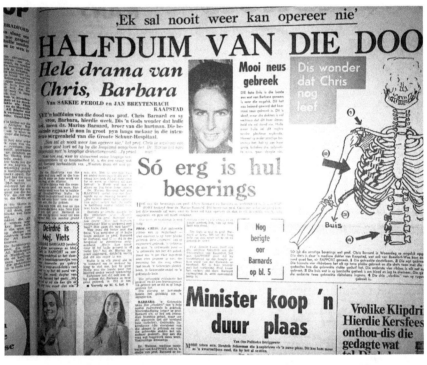

The front page of a Sunday paper on the morning after the hit-and-run
incident. The arrows indicate the injuries Barnard sustained.

CHAPTER 14

Rumours of assassination

THE MISSIONARY'S SON FROM THE KAROO REMAINED OPPOSED TO apartheid. It couldn't be any other way. Christiaan Barnard used every platform he was given to criticise the government's racist laws and he slammed ongoing racial discrimination wherever he went. Still, he remained a loyal South African and turned down multiple offers of better employment at institutions that were much better resourced than Groote Schuur.

His antagonism towards the Nationalist Party (NP) and its apartheid ideology of racial segregation had its roots in Beaufort West, where he had experienced some of the worst discrimination first hand as the son of a missionary who tended to the coloured community in a deeply divided town. His feelings deepened at university, where he voiced his opposition to the discrimination shown towards black, coloured and Indian doctors who were all paid less than their white colleagues with the same education. Medicine would always consume the bulk of Barnard's time but his vocal opposition to apartheid never stopped and was reported widely following the heart transplant.

In one instance, on 21 April 1969, Barnard got into trouble with his bosses for daring to criticise the ongoing pay disparity between black and white doctors in South Africa.[1]

This was but one example. His continued criticism of a government consisting of largely fellow Afrikaners did not go unnoticed and had some big personal implications, one of which was that he started getting death threats after the heart transplant.

although I am aware of
the difficulties con fronting the government
in this matter, it is my
personal view that it is wrong
to pay doctors less because they
are not White, although they are
equally qualified and do the
same work as their White colleague
    I urge the government to give
assurances that they will narrow
the present gap steadily and
progressively.
    I believe that we can achieve this,
but the best way to do so is for
our non-White colleagues not to resign
to continue at their posts, serving their
patients and their country.

In this handwritten note Barnard expresses his views on pay
discrimination between doctors based on race.

'I never took the death threats seriously, except maybe one time. The time and place of the attack was too well planned.'

Barnard had been invited to Oudtshoorn, which included a visit to the famous Cango Caves. An anonymous letter writer knew Chris's itinerary and warned that 'when the lights dim, you will be killed'.

'I tried not to concern myself with it but the police took it quite seriously and provided me with bodyguards. We entered the caves and reached the spot where the lights dimmed. My guards moved in closer. When the lights went on again, I shifted to my left but no-one tried to kill me. When we got outside again the one policeman said, "I told you there was nothing to worry about," but I couldn't help but notice he was sweating heavily just like me and his hand was shaking lightly as he lit his cigarette.'

Barnard's continued criticism of the government possibly led to an actual assassination attempt in December 1972, which nearly succeeded. There is no clear evidence of a firm plan to kill the famous doctor but following all the clues, the conclusion is not too far-fetched.

Warnings

In Cape Town during a business dinner, Barnard angered the Nationalists when he said that he needed help with some answers because he kept getting asked the same questions on his travels.

'In Denmark, they ask why we allow black and coloured women to look after our children and care for them in our homes but we won't allow them to care for our patients in our hospitals.'

Barnard's comments quickly turned the crowd against him but he pressed on.

Many of the attendees started getting up and leaving the dinner with some shouting loudly that Barnard was making a fool of himself.

'I cannot answer these questions, so please help me out,' Barnard told the dwindling audience, as he called for a more progressive South Africa.

He repeated that his political sympathies were not with the NP.[2]

In response, the Afrikaans media went for Barnard, as they always did when it came to his political leanings. *Die Transvaler* and *Die Vaderland* newspapers, which were considered to be pro-NP, lashed out at Barnard and warned him to stay away from politics. *Die Transvaler* stated that it was noticeable that Barnard's private life was 'colourful for a doctor' and that this was tolerated but that Barnard's political statements would not be treated in the same fashion.

'If he wishes to keep the respect of the public, he will stay away from politics and the political terrain,' the newspaper warned.

On 8 November 1969, Barnard reacted to the continued criticism of his own anti-government statements and said that extreme right-wing policies posed a greater risk to South Africa's white population than did communism.

'As a doctor, it's my duty to treat suffering, and human suffering [from oppression], I consider to be far worse than the physical suffering of a man with heart disease.'

Again, Barnard repeated how ridiculous racial segregation actually was. 'What right does the South African government have to state that Japanese people are whites and Chinese people are coloured? What is that based on?'[3]

His comments to a crowd of Johannesburg businessmen in 1970 were even more fiery. The people attending were mostly members of the Broederbond and when Barnard stood at the podium to deliver his keynote address, he said the title of his speech was 'Why we deserve to be called Nazis'.

Before he could be stopped, he explained the similarities between apartheid legislation and the legislation that Nazi Germany had implemented to limit the freedoms of the Jews.

'The Nationalists issued the Group Areas Act to limit black, coloured and Indian people to certain areas. The Nazis shoved the Jews into ghettos. In South Africa, some positions are for whites only. In Nazi Germany, Jews were prevented from certain positions. In South Africa, there are signs everywhere stating "whites only". In Nazi Germany it was "Juden verboten".'

Barnard warned the audience that there should be no surprise if outsiders were vehemently opposed to South Africa when white South Africans kept trying to drive the perception that they were a superior race, while the world saw how inhumanely their fellow countrymen were treated.

Nico Malan, the Administrator of the Cape Province, and National Government cabinet ministers contacted Barnard and lambasted him for his statements.

'I was accused of being un-Christian and politically naïve.'

On 15 December 1970, Barnard stood together with a group of prominent South Africans who threatened to boycott the new Nico Malan Theatre in Cape Town. They were unhappy with plans to exclude coloured and black people from the theatre. The theatre was initially meant to be managed in accordance with apartheid legislation, which would have had this effect.

'I could have remained the blue-eyed boy of the government if I'd wanted to and if I'd kept quiet and accepted things as they were. I could have been the Minister of Health, but then I wouldn't have been able to live with myself,' Barnard said.

Professional boycott

The first action taken against Barnard targeted him professionally. By April 1971, heart transplants across the world were in decline. The rest of the world was becoming increasingly worried about the bad outcomes of these operations, as most patients were dying soon after they received new hearts. Barnard, however, never doubted that the procedure was a viable mechanism to treat patients with no other options.

He became increasingly convinced that doctors in South Africa no longer wanted to send him patients for heart transplants and he stated that these doctors preferred to send patients home to die than to refer them to him.[4]

There is some truth in this. Dirk van Zyl was Barnard's first transplant patient in two years. One Sunday newspaper even commented that Barnard was being boycotted. Such a boycott would have made no sense unless it was personal or political in nature, because Barnard's results in contrast to the global results were excellent. By this time his fifth patient, Dorothy Fischer, had already been living for two years after her procedure.

On 24 April 1971, Barnard addressed a room full of people at the second anniversary of Fischer's transplant. She was at this stage the longest living survivor of a heart transplant. The celebration was held at the Mount Nelson Hotel in central Cape Town and was attended by mainly black and coloured people. Such was the nature of apartheid legislation that the organisers had to get special permission from the government to hold the multiracial gathering. Barnard was the keynote speaker and he said that he and his team were quite comfortable at a multiracial gathering.

'Surgeons work on the inside of people, and on the inside all people are the same,' Barnard stated.

He complained again that doctors were no longer sending him patients and said that if the status quo continued, he would not be able to continue with his work in Cape Town and may have to leave.[5] During this speech, he was overcome with emotion and couldn't finish.

Between December 1967 and May 1971, Barnard performed six heart transplants. The patients were Washkansky (survived 18 days), Blaiberg (593 days), Petrus Smith (622 days), Douglas Killops (64 days), Dorothy Fischer (4 568 days) and Dirk van Zyl (8 458 days).

The average survival rate for these six patients was six and a half years, with Van Zyl going on to live for 23 years with his second heart. In contrast, the rest of the world's record was atrocious. Only 18% of all patients were surviving for longer than one year. Barnard's record was unsurpassed.

Journalist Bob Molloy wrote later that Barnard's outspokenness did not go unpunished.

'He always expressed strong anti-apartheid sentiments in each public speech and was always ready with a comment to criticise the govern-ment. The authorities reacted. His fall from grace was seen in the small things. He had always received red-carpet treatment at places like air-ports. This was cancelled, as well as other privileges, including the use of private suites and assistance with customs when he was travelling. Airport officials would simply shrug and state that the orders had come from above.'

Marius Barnard

In South Africa, 1972 was a year of unrest. Residents of informal set-tlements were angry and standing up against the apartheid government which, in turn, started to use increasingly violent means to quash the unrest and keep people in check.

On 7 June 1972, Marius Barnard addressed a gathering of student protestors at the Cape Town City Hall, where he spoke out about the need to improve education for black people. Afrikaners were angry and lashed out at Marius, despite his involvement in the heart transplant in 1967. One moment he was a golden child and the next he was hated. Beaufort West's mayor even stated that he was embarrassed by the fact that Chris and Marius Barnard had been born in the town.

Marius was warned that he would be charged for addressing the anti-apartheid student protest and making statements against the gov-ernment. He was told that he was in danger of losing his job. Chris immediately announced that if his brother lost his job, he would resign and leave with Marius.[6]

Shortly after this, Chris was in trouble again after being quoted in *Die Burger*. He had addressed a gathering of the Western Cape Blood Transfusion Services and said that 6% of the children that he and his team treated, died after they returned home.[7]

'Most of them [the children who died] are coloured and black chil-dren who we must send out of the hospital to shanty towns where they die of malnutrition or lung disease. They die despite the hard work, thousands of rand invested doing intricate operations and lots of love poured out on them in the hospital. Sometimes one wonders if it wouldn't be better to simply cut their throats,' Barnard said.[8]

Calling for regime change

It was the final straw when, on 25 November 1972, Chris Barnard was unequivocal.

'I believe a regime change is necessary in South Africa,' he is quoted as saying in *The New York Times*.

The newspaper was quoting from an interview Barnard had done in Cape Town in which he said that he had joined the opposition political party, the United Party (UP), and would be standing for Parliament in opposition to the NP. Barnard said that his brother Marius might also stand as an 'anti-government candidate'.

The *Sunday Times* quoted Barnard as saying that 'the Nationalist government had to be ousted in the best interests of South Africa'. He said that South Africa could no longer stand by a government whose only tune was the racial one.

Die Transvaler came out against Barnard, making it clear that he was in danger of losing his job at the government hospital, Groote Schuur.[9]

Tremendous pressure was put on the Barnards through multiple media platforms and a rumour was spread that there was to be an official investigation into their political activities.

Sunday newspapers reported that Barnard was 'abusing his position to attack the government'. Again, the brothers' hometown spared them no pain and the local media reiterated the message that the town was sorry that the Barnards had been born there. There were multiple accounts of Afrikaners in the area who felt betrayed by the brothers who had joined the UP.

'They are making it quite clear that they don't want me back in my hometown, but they needn't be worried, I will never go back again,' Chris stated.

He said he could recall how his father, Adam, had fought for decades against the town's plans to have his coloured congregation and school moved out of the town.

'When my dad wasn't there any more, the congregation was moved. The church is no longer a church, instead it was turned into a badminton hall. I will never go back there again,' Chris stated.

On the 12 December 1972, Barnard stated, amid growing pressure and calls for his resignation, that he would never resign voluntarily. 'I have hundreds of patients who rely on me.'

What happened next was quite astounding.

Hit and run

A day later, on 13 December 1972, Chris Barnard and his 22-year-old wife Barbara left their favourite Italian restaurant in Sea Point. They were crossing the road when out of the blue a bakkie accelerated towards them and hit them. Some eyewitnesses stated that the bakkie had been parked at the side of the road and had pulled out very quickly.

Chris and Barbara were flung through the air. Chris initially slammed into his wife, which probably saved his life. Barbara, in turn, landed on a parked car, which probably prevented her from breaking her neck.

The bakkie raced off.

A motorist who had seen what had happened raced after the bakkie but lost it in traffic.[10] All the motorist could register was a portion of a number plate. It started with CZ – the registration for Beaufort West.

The Barnards were rushed to hospital in a serious condition and Marius Barnard and Rodney Hewitson were called in.

'I kept asking about Barbara. They kept saying she hadn't been badly hurt. I couldn't know that she had been seriously injured and but for the grace of God she hadn't died. Several of her neck vertebrae were broken and her left shoulder blade was crushed,' Chris wrote later.

Chris was seriously injured, with possible bleeding on one kidney and multiple broken bones, including several broken ribs. Marius spent the night next to his brother's bed.

'It's a miracle that they survived,' Marius said.

'What happened?' Chris wanted to know.

'From what we hear, it was a hit and run,' Marius explained.

He continued: 'Some say it could even have been politically motivated because there was apparently a car waiting outside the restaurant. When you left, it pulled away suddenly, ran you over and raced off.'

Marius explained that Barbara had been lucky that she had fallen on the parked car or she might well have died.

Barbara's accident left her with irreparable nerve damage, which included limiting the use of her left hand due to the shoulder damage. She was unable to lift her left hand above her shoulder for the rest of her life.

'Whenever she had to use this hand – for example, when she had to do her hair – she would use the other hand to prop the left hand into position. Most often no-one even noticed,' friend Don Mackenzie remembers.[11]

Chris broke eight ribs on his right-hand side and cracked three vertebrae.

The public believed that the accident had been an attempted assassination by Barnard's opponents as a result of his ongoing anti-apartheid criticism. His public announcement about his political aspirations and joining the opposition UP, and the accompanying media reports and warnings, fuelled this speculation.

It was acknowledged in the press that there was little substance to the theory of attempted assassination but it certainly became evident that most South Africans believed their foremost surgeon could have been the subject of an attempted assassination.

On 14 December, a 27-year-old man, Kallie Lufele, was arrested in connection with the hit-and-run accident, but the state had to release him again on 30 January when no evidence could be found that he had been involved. The culprits were never found.

Barnard spent three weeks recovering in hospital.

Withdrawal from politics

Six months after the accident, Chris Barnard announced that he was withdrawing from active politics and had let go of his political aspirations. He said that he had changed his mind because he had become despondent about politics, and that he would focus in future on the operating table.[12] He chose not to expand on the reasons for his despondency.[13]

Marius Barnard eventually resigned from Groote Schuur Hospital in 1980 and went to Parliament as a member of the opposition Progressive Federal Party (PFP) as MP for Parktown. Chris never entered active politics.

The full extent of the impact of the hit and run on Chris Barnard is impossible to determine. It certainly seems, however, that it led to him adopting a different strategy in taking on the government going forward.

In 1993 Barnard wrote about his own struggle as follows: 'The knowledge that I should have done more kept haunting me. I should actually have become a terrorist, I told myself. But I wasn't. Like others, I only did enough to soothe my conscience but not enough to cause trouble. We were cowards who cared for our own safety and comfort above all else. Of course, we could offer excuses – I had my family and children to consider. Whenever I could, I spoke out against apartheid but what did we really do to bring about the fall of the South African government? Nothing except not voting NP. How courageous. Sadly, many people started accepting that I was working for the regime while, instead, I was using the system against itself.'[14]

Was there an attempt to kill Christiaan Barnard? We shall never know for sure – not while the identity of that hit-and-run driver remains a secret.

Barbara had always been superstitious and she had had a little mantra she would repeat when she saw a passing ambulance. It went like this: 'touch your head, touch your toes, I hope I never go in one of those.' After the accident, she never uttered it again.[15]

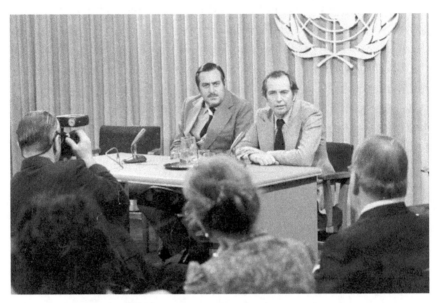

*Pik Botha and Chris Barnard addressing the media in the
media room at the United Nations.*

PHOTOGRAPH WITH PERMISSION OF PIK BOTHA.

CHAPTER 15

Politics

IN THE EYES OF THE WORLD CHRISTIAAN BARNARD COULD DO NO WRONG. Doors were opened and the red carpet rolled out wherever he went. He was the miracle man, the charming, brilliant doctor from Cape Town. Barnard met with world leaders in their palaces and their private homes. His life became one of fantasy and glamour, far removed from the dirt roads of the Karoo.

Once, when Barbara and Chris were visiting the Philippines, they were invited on the spur of the moment to attend the coronation of the new king of Nepal in Kathmandu.

'My passport won't allow me to enter Nepal,' Barnard said.[1]

The Philippine leader, Ferdinand Marcos, promptly gave the Barnards honorary Philippine citizenship and had them issued with passports, thereby enabling them to attend the coronation.

Chris Barnard was still making public statements against the government from time to time, despite his near-death experience.

In 1974, he petitioned the state to release Bram Fischer, the Afrikaner lawyer who had defended the Rivonia trialists, including Nelson Mandela, against treason charges. Fischer had been jailed for life on communism charges in 1966. While in jail, he was diagnosed with cancer and became increasingly sick. Barnard's pleas fell on deaf ears, with Prime Minister John Vorster stating, 'Stay out of politics and I will stay out of the operating theatre.'

Fischer died in 1975, a few weeks after being moved to his brother's house.

The state would not leave Barnard alone. He had become too much of an asset, despite his ongoing criticism. As the heart surgeon's image bloomed, South Africa's image on the global stage dimmed. Anti-apartheid activism, including increasingly severe boycotts, and other economic sanctions started to bite. One real problem for the state was that communication channels were all closing and the country was getting increasingly isolated. With official channels failing and doors shutting everywhere, it became increasingly difficult for the South African government to reach out to other world leaders.

'Ambassadors couldn't achieve anything. No-one wanted to listen to us, no-one wanted to talk to us,' says the ex-Minister of Foreign Affairs, Pik Botha.

For a country whose economy was still dependent on foreign markets and desperately needed commodities like oil, this situation was disastrous. Accordingly, a project was started under the Department of Information, a project that became known as the Information Scandal. An estimated R75 million was spent on this covert propaganda operation. The money came from secret slush funds in the secret budgets of the Ministry of Defence headed by a certain Minister PW Botha.[2]

The aim of the project was to improve South Africa's global image, by among other things, buying – and controlling – English-language newspapers. At that stage, the Afrikaans media were considered to be less of a threat.

The person in charge of this project was Dr Eschel Rhoodie, an attractive dark-haired man, considered to be enlightened and brilliant. He understood that the state needed to develop new ways of communicating with the outside world.

At the time, there were two South Africans who were welcomed with open arms across the world, despite the apartheid state's increasingly pariah status. They were Barnard and the star golfer Gary Player. Barnard and Player's public image on the world stage was welcome relief for the apartheid state, but it made them targets for the state's own goals.

The state started using Barnard's success to polish the country's image at a time when the world was condemning anything South African.[3]

Kobus Visser, Barnard's son-in-law, says the situation could be best explained as follows: 'It wasn't going well for the state in those days. Apartheid could simply not be defended and to take the spotlight off apartheid and refocus it elsewhere – on something like Chris Barnard – was ideal. The state started using him as a lightning conductor.'

Ambassador

Pik Botha says Barnard helped to keep some communication channels open with foreign states.

'He was the brilliant doctor who had transplanted the first heart. I was a career politician. The world attacked me with glee. Not many people took him on. All the while, Chris never defended apartheid and was certainly no racist. Sometimes he lost his temper and when he lost his temper he was difficult. But he was a human being, like all of us.'

Botha says that Barnard helped him understand that for real change to come to South Africa, it was important that people who shared the same values band together and stand together, regardless of race or background.

'Chris saw the larger picture and understood what the impact of complete sanctions and boycotts on South Africa would mean. The goal of such total sanctions was the complete economic destruction of South Africa. Chris realised that that would hit the poorest the hardest.'

Botha says Barnard was also not in favour of the regime.

'He simply realised that if we became economically crippled, the entire country would be stuffed. While he never acted in favour of apartheid, he acted against world forces that wanted to destroy South Africa completely, thereby affecting all South Africans. He was also opposed to people who insisted everyone in South Africa was racist. At the end of the day, Chris didn't want his country to be destroyed. He was never pro-apartheid but he was always pro-South Africa.'

'I'm not a politician, I'm a doctor who can only treat patients that I come into touch with. Touchpoints are places where pressure can be

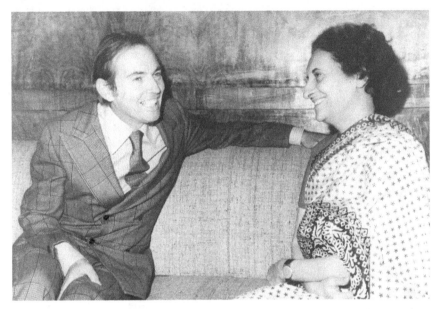

The Prime Minister of India, Indira Gandhi, and Chris Barnard. Barnard was no fan
of Gandhi's, claiming she was suppressing opposition politicians and the press.

PHOTOGRAPH COURTESY OF THE HEART OF CAPE TOWN MUSEUM

applied and South Africa needs pressure to get rid of apartheid,' Barnard
wrote.

Still, his politics and outspokenness got him into trouble. In 1977, he
caused a stir with the publication of a book called *South Africa: Sharp
Dissection*. In this book, he called on the South African government
to do away with all discriminatory laws and to implement a one-man,
one-vote system for the election of a government. The book was, under-
standably, not well received locally.

It was also not well received outside South Africa because Barnard
lashed out at the 'political hypocrisy' in the world, stating that there
were many countries similar to South Africa where similar discriminatory racial policies were in effect and where there were many limits to
freedoms, including speech and politics. He highlighted, as an example,
India under Indira Gandhi and questioned the banning of political parties and jailing of hundreds of opposition political activists.

'She was locking up journalists and editors and closing down the free press, but all she wanted to speak about was how terrible South Africa was.'

Barnard echoed Botha's sentiment: 'The world doesn't understand that being pro-South Africa does not mean being pro-apartheid.'

Robert Sobukwe

In June 1977, Robert Sobukwe, a prominent South African political dissident and founder of the Pan Africanist Congress (PAC), told his friend, newspaperman Benjamin Pogrund, during their regular telephonic conversations, that he was feeling unwell.[4]

The apartheid regime had Sobukwe under house arrest in Kimberley after six years of imprisonment on Robben Island, where he had been kept in isolation. Sobukwe started complaining of fever and developed a bad cough. A specialist in Johannesburg diagnosed cancer in Sobukwe's lung. An urgent operation was needed.[5]

The state wanted to send Sobukwe to Bloemfontein for treatment but the PAC leader refused and insisted on being sent to Cape Town – to Groote Schuur, where the Barnards were.

'[Chris] Barnard – himself an Afrikaner – was the opposite of the stereotypical image of Afrikaners and would provide invaluable support to Sobukwe,' Pogrund recalls.[6]

Eight years and six months after his release from prison, Sobukwe returned to Cape Town, a very sick man.[7]

Marius Barnard remembers that Sobukwe arrived at the hospital together with a large contingent of security police.[8] When Sobukwe arrived, Chris was overseas. Two other members of the medical team, doctors Joe de Nobrega and Rodney Hewitson, would play a huge role in Sobukwe's treatment.

'Joe was a registrar in thoracic surgery. Previously he had been a centre forward for the Cape Town football team Cape Town City. Everyone loved Joe. He was an excellent doctor and showed a great interest in the treatment of the new patient,' according to Marius.[9]

Pogrund recalls that Sobukwe's lung was removed on Wednesday, 14 September, two days after he was admitted to Groote Schuur. 'Hewitson, probably the best chest specialist in the country, did the operation.'[10]

'Sobukwe got the best treatment Groote Schuur had to offer,' De Nobrega confirms.[11]

During the operation, Hewitson found that the cancer had already spread.

'He removed the lung and this was to be followed by three weeks of recovery to allow the wound to heal. Thereafter Sobukwe had to receive radiotherapy treatment. Sobukwe went through a difficult, slow and painful recovery,' says Marius.[12]

The medical staff were impressed by Sobukwe.

'We nursed him in a single, private room. There were always two security policemen at the door.'[13]

Shortly after the operation, Chris Barnard returned to Groote Schuur where he was informed about the new patient.

He recalls this moment rather forcefully in his later memoirs: 'The NP government had carte blanche in those days and were banning organisations and locking up their leaders. Most white people did nothing. Why should we get involved? Life is good, everything is comfortable and there's no need to make things complicated. We were all living an easy life. So we accepted the way things were, besides a few voices calling in the wilderness, and looked the other way.'[14]

Chris was still the boss and immediately took control of Sobukwe's care. He acted with great empathy towards him and instructed the staff to make sure the patient was as comfortable as possible.[15] One of his first steps was to get rid of the security police.

'When he discovered Sobukwe was in our ward, he chased the security police away and said the patient was his responsibility and that he would not allow anything that could compromise Sobukwe's recovery. The men were shocked but they removed themselves speedily,' Marius recalls.

De Nobrega says Barnard chased the security police away 'as though they were 12-year-old schoolboys. They had to spend the rest of their time there in the hospital's parking lot.'[16]

Pogrund also recalls Barnard's role in this positive light.

'Initially Sobukwe was under 24-hour watch, with the two guards always close. These guards ordered the doctors to prevent all visitors except direct family. [Chris] Barnard then arrived and said, "This is my ward and I take the responsibility for my patients," and then he chased them out.'[17]

Chris grabbed the opportunity and held long talks with Sobukwe when possible. He wanted to discover first hand from one of the leaders of a black consciousness movement what their wishes and aspirations were.

'He was a dying man but still believed that he would live to see the day when the country would be free from the unholy influence of apartheid. I spent hours with him and tried my best to relieve his suffering. We allowed him to leave the hospital over weekends but even this small gesture was limited by the unsympathetic security machine of the state. When I told the police on duty he was a dying man who couldn't harm anyone, they said I should stick to medicine and they would look after the safety of the state. The commander insisted Sobukwe was dangerous and that the house arrest order had to be strictly adhered to. Robert accepted the humiliation with grace and bore the suffering without complaint.'[18]

'He knew about me and we enjoyed many discussions. He was a deeply religious man and his wife Veronica – the most wonderful woman – visited him twice daily. They were often observed reading together from the Bible. Sobukwe had a magnetic personality. Once you were with him you were under the impression this was a wonderful person. It was remarkable to note that he showed no hatred or bitterness,' Marius remembers.[19]

Helen Suzman also visited Sobukwe in hospital. 'At our last meeting, he was terminal and close to the end. I was touched by his lack of bitterness towards a wasted life that was coming to an end. He was sad and unhappy about the deterioration of race relations in the country.'[20]

During this period, Chris Barnard went to Pretoria to meet with Prime Minister John Vorster, hoping that there was something more that could be done for Sobukwe.

'After I told him about my conversations with Sobukwe, Mr Vorster agreed to meet with him too and asked me to make the arrangements. I was very excited and couldn't wait to deliver the good news to my patient. I ran up the stairs to his room and said, "Robert, I'm bringing good news. I spoke to the Prime Minister and he has agreed to meet with you." Sobukwe's face darkened and he stated he had nothing to say to Vorster. "I will speak to him when he is ready to give the country to me." He lay back in his bed, subject closed.'

De Nobrega, who was in charge of the ward, offered to house the Sobukwes at his home for the three weeks he was to receive the radio-therapy treatment.

Pogrund remembers the De Nobregas.

'Joe's wife, Nita, was also a doctor. They weren't interested in politics given their long working hours but they knew who Sobukwe was.'[21]

The offer was made and accepted, and Sobukwe and his wife spent three weeks in the home of the De Nobregas in Oranjezicht.

'I had to carry him up and down the stairs every day, he was so weak. He enjoyed sitting in the sun and we had many conversations in those days. He was hugely intelligent and we discussed everything and any-thing. He was happy and comfortable to recover in that environment. One day I asked him if he'd like to go for a ride and he said he'd like to go to Signal Hill. He wanted to see Robben Island again.'

When his treatment was completed, the Sobukwes returned to Kimberley, where Robert died in the Kimberley General Hospital on 27 February 1978. Veronica was by his side.

The Sobukwe children were living in the United States at the time with the American ambassador to the United Nations, Andrew Young. Barnard called Young and asked if he was going to send the three chil-dren home to attend their father's funeral.

'He said there wasn't enough money to do that so I made some plans to get the money together,' Barnard later recalled.

Barnard went to his government contacts and demanded money for the air tickets from New York to South Africa.

'The day that Sobukwe died, Barnard offered Veronica the R4 000 the children needed for their flights. I recommended that she take it and she did,' Pogrund recalls.[22]

'Mrs Sobukwe called me later and thanked me for the arrangements. No-one knew where the money came from. My time with Sobukwe had left a lasting impression. I was saddened to hear of his death,' Barnard wrote.[23]

Barnard's help for the Sobukwe children came at a cost. When Eschel Rhoodie appeared in court in The Hague, shortly after being arrested overseas on fraud charges, he explained: 'Barnard's biggest role was when he helped to convince the American Trade Union leader George Meaney to not support a call for a global trade-union boycott against South Africa.'[24]

Rhoodie said that Barnard had agreed to meet with Meaney only once he had 'been given assurances that the Sobukwe children could attend their father's funeral without fear of arrest or intimidation'.[25]

Barnard's meeting with Meaney helped to prevent a global boycott of all sea and air shipping routes to South Africa.

'The impact of that could not be measured in monetary terms. But even a week's blockade would have cost South Africa hundreds of millions of rand. So I made sure that there were no stumbling blocks in Chris's path to bring the Sobukwe children to South Africa. He flew at our expense from Boston to Washington to meet Meaney.'

Joe and Nita de Nobrega attended Sobukwe's funeral in Graaff-Reinet, where he had been born.

Breyten Breytenbach

As was the case with Bram Fischer, Barnard took on the state again over its treatment of another prominent Afrikaner struggle activist, the poet Breyten Breytenbach.

Breyten was arrested in 1975 because he had entered South Africa on a fake French passport under a false name. He had lived in Paris for more than 15 years and was married to a Vietnamese woman, which also

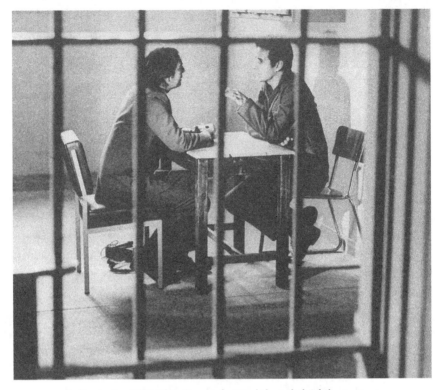

In December 1977 Chris Barnard visited the jailed Afrikaans poet
Breyten Breytenbach in Pollsmoor Prison. Barnard would plead for
Breytenbach's release from jail, but to no avail.

© GALLO IMAGES / HUISGENOOT

posed problems because marriages across the colour line had been illegal in South Africa since 1949.

Breytenbach was charged on 11 counts under the Terrorism Act and the Suppression of Communism Act. These charges included arms smuggling, the planning of sabotage, spying on harbours and conspiracy. Surprisingly, Breytenbach pleaded guilty – perhaps to taunt the state – and was sentenced to nine years in prison, the greater part of which would be served in solitary confinement.

Barnard said that the civil service at the time was staffed primarily by Afrikaners so Breytenbach could have expected to be treated worse than most prisoners because Afrikaners considered him to be a traitor.

On a visit to France in 1977, Barnard was peppered with questions about Breytenbach's condition in South Africa's prisons.

On his return, he managed to arrange a visit to Breytenbach in Pollsmoor Prison – he wanted to ascertain the welfare of the poet. This was on 23 December 1977, two days before Christmas. He took a French television crew along with him. The meeting was also reported in the Afrikaans magazine, *Huisgenoot*, which carried several photographs under the headline 'Prof Chris with Breyten in Cell'. In the black-and-white photographs, the two men can be seen seated opposite each other at a table, steel bars in the foreground.[26]

Barnard's interview with Breytenbach was broadcast on French television.

'He [Breytenbach] was clearly happy to see the professor and said that his intention had never been to overthrow the South African Government with violence. The television interview lasted eight minutes,' stated the article.[27]

After the interview, Barnard was quite shaken by Breytenbach's circumstances.

'My heart goes out to this sensitive, polite man who had become the sacrifice of circumstances. It's sad to see how he is being emotionally broken down by the rough and unmannered jailors for whom he must always address "Yes, Sir, no, Sir". The same jailors lambasted me for addressing him with respect. For them he is simply "Breytenbach".[28]

Barnard went to see Vorster again and pleaded for the release of Breytenbach since he was no threat to South Africa.

'He refused.'

Breytenbach's own recollections of his meeting with Barnard are written up in his 1984 memoir, *The True Confessions of an Albino Terrorist*. In this he refers to Barnard as Christ Barnard, the heart plumber.

'I was summoned to the VIP visiting room in Cape Town one afternoon and, to my astonishment, left quite alone without any supervision in the presence of this doctor. He was very friendly and wanted to know if I would participate in a film he was making about South Africa for

French television. Everything had already been arranged with the prison department, he said. Again, then the iniquitous choice one is faced with: the possibility, however faint, of communicating with the outside world (and remember that the filming would in any event be a break in the rotting away rott of everyday life in prison), but at the same time it could be a trick to use one for propaganda purposes. I asked for permission to consult my lawyers before making any decision and this was granted. I wanted them to look into the project and see if it was really on the level.'[29]

Breytenbach heard nothing from his lawyers and a few weeks passed before he was fetched in an almighty rush one afternoon and taken to the general prison stores.

'I was to prepare myself immediately for the filming because the professor and the French crew were already on their way. But I hadn't heard anything from my lawyers, I objected. "Very strange", he clucked in sympathy. "They can't be very serious about their work, can they now, because we have forwarded your letter."'[30]

Later Breytenbach found out that his lawyers had never been contacted by the authorities.

'I should have known better, or been stronger but I allowed myself to be bamboozled into the farce. Striding with legs wide apart, they took me to the section store where our clothes were kept and an underling ran over to the female prison at the double with a brand-new outfit over his arm, to have it pressed. The TV crew turned up. They wanted to film me in my cell. The warden had arranged for a bedspread to be thrown over my bed and wanted to bring in a carpet too but I objected to these foolish attempts at masking the bareness. Barnard then proceeded to interview me. Whenever there was a break in the filming he would switch off his recorder and say to me softly, you know I agree entirely with your views. I don't like this government either. I support you wholeheartedly. And when the cameraman was ready for the next take he would go back to his mouthings of pro South African propaganda.'[31]

Breytenbach writes that Barnard visited him in jail twice more.

'I must grant that these were pleasant occasions – except that I could never get a word in edgeways. These were also contact visits and of the red-carpet variety, the sort my wife and father never received. Still, in his tortured way, he did sincerely attempt to put in a good word for me.'[32]

Barnard approached the Minister of Police, Jimmy Kruger, and asked for Breytenbach's release, but the minister also refused.

Eighteen months after Barnard met with Breytenbach for the first time in his cell, Kruger yet again refused the poet parole. Barnard responded in a column in the *Cape Times*, under the title 'I Mourn with You', as follows:

'The Minister of Police announced the decision but the silence of Afrikanerdom blessed it. One day, when we look back at this silent blessing we will see it for what it actually was: a curse on Afrikanerdom by Afrikaners.'

Barnard wrote about the poet he had found in hell; the hell of a man whose spirit was dying in isolation.

'How did it come to this? Do we have so much fear that we are scared to release a poet?'[33]

The Information Scandal

Rhoodie and Barnard were in touch for about six years during which they became friends socially – both were notorious party animals.

Connie Mulder, the father of Dr Pieter Mulder, the ex-leader of the opposition political party, the Freedom Front Plus, was also part of the inner circle in the NP Government at the time, and was also involved in the Information Scandal.

Pieter Mulder said that the state's secret propaganda projects covered a period of roughly 10 years.

'My dad explained later that Eschel Rhoodie realised that if the propaganda war was lost, the next step was a militarisation. Following the leaks of the Information Scandal, that is precisely what happened. The country became increasingly militaristic and even developed nuclear weapons under PW Botha.'[34]

Only three people were held accountable for the Information Scandal

– Eschel Rhoodie, Connie Mulder and John Vorster. Following the leaks and after the fallout, PW Botha became the leader of the NP.

Barnard was not implicated because he had duly accounted for every cent he had been reimbursed by the state when he was on official business that cost him money.

'At one stage I had believed it was possible to change the Government's thinking by means of subtle convincing and I kept at it for some time. I was wrong. The Government had been in the saddle for too long and had become so arrogant and dictatorial that there was no way such an approach would have worked.'[35]

Steve Biko

Correspondence at the Beaufort West Museum shows how Barnard got involved with a handful of doctors who wanted to take action against their colleagues, whom they felt had failed in their duty towards Steve Biko.

Doctors who had treated Biko had observed his condition after he had received several beatings and had failed to act to save him. Some in the profession wanted action taken against these doctors and instituted a legal campaign against the South African Medical and Dental Council for not acting against the guilty doctors.

Dr Frances Ames was one of the leaders in this action. In August 1980 she wrote to Barnard: 'Apparently my word about your word is not enough. Could you send me a letter saying that you are prepared publicly to support a move to take legal action against the Medical and Dental Council in regard to the Biko affair? Your support will be invaluable.'[36]

In reaction, Barnard instructed his lawyer, Noel Tunbridge, as follows: 'A group of doctors which includes me, feel that this case should be lodged with the Supreme Court.'[37]

Barnard retired before the case finally went to the Supreme Court eight years later where it would end in victory for Ames and her colleagues.

Barnard's politics was complex but there can be no doubt that he was no racist and staunchly opposed to apartheid and the NP. In his own way, he did what he could at the time but it would always haunt him that he should have done more.

In later years, when he heard that Barnard had died, Nelson Mandela said, 'His death is a great loss for the country after all the contributions he made. He was one of South Africa's main achievers who has also done very well in expressing his opinion on apartheid.'

PART FOUR

How to fall and get up again, 1983–2001

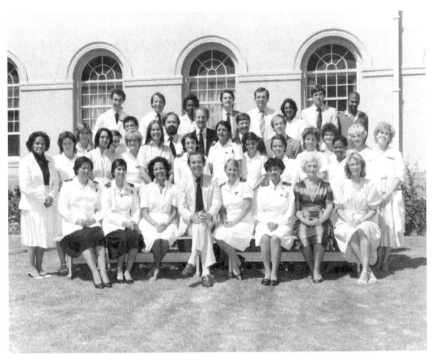

*Staff from the surgery department and transplant teams at
Groote Schuur on the last day of Chris Barnard's employment,
December 1983. He retired aged 61, suffering from rheumatoid arthritis.
He was gifted for his years of service – with a tie.*

PHOTOGRAPH COURTESY OF THE HEART OF CAPE TOWN MUSEUM

CHAPTER 16

Retirement, tragedy and scandal

E ARLY ONE MORNING IN 1981, THE TELEPHONE STARTED RINGING ON the bedside table in the Stanford Court Hotel in San Francisco. Chris Barnard was in America to promote his latest book, *The Body Machine*, which he had co-authored.

Barbara had become the owner of a successful boutique clothing store called BnB in Cape Town's Golden Acre shopping centre. She was famous for her fantastic fashion shows. Like her famous husband, she didn't hesitate to show the government's segregationist policies a middle finger and always insisted on using black models.[1]

Barnard picked up the phone. 'Chris Barnard.'

'I have bad news.' It was Noel Tunbridge, Chris's lawyer, calling from South Africa. 'Barbara wants a divorce.'

'Why?' is all Barnard could get out.

'According to Barbara, your domestic helpers discovered you in bed with another woman a few weeks ago when Barbara was overseas buying outfits for her shop.'[2]

Once again in San Francisco, Barnard's romantic life had come full circle – this was where he and Louwtjie had seen their relationship derail spectacularly.

His long trail of broken hearts and sexual conquests had continued over the years, despite his marriage to Barbara. For a while he had got away with it. But no longer.

Back in South Africa, Chris tried to explain it all away with yet another story: 'I was in bed with a cold. A young woman and her friend came to visit and later the friend left. The girl stayed a while longer to chat. There is no truth in the story that we slept together.'

But Barbara didn't believe him. 'Both helpers told me, Chris. Both of them.'

Barbara kicked Chris out of the house. She'd had enough.

Once again, the heart pioneer was left holding a bag of clothes, without a roof over his head.

On 13 January 1982, a month before the couple would have celebrated their 12th wedding anniversary, the marriage ended in divorce in the Cape Town High Court. The Barnards had two young sons at the time, Frederick and Christiaan junior.

For some time, Chris blamed his arthritis and age, and remained convinced that they had played a large part in Barbara's decision.

'Barbara met a younger man, one who could offer her the sort of life I never could.'[3]

One Sunday afternoon, when Chris was dropping off the two boys at Barbara's home, he ran into the new man who was 'walking around in a speedo as if he owned the place'.

For the next six months Chris Barnard was consumed by jealousy.

'I had a tremendous emotional reaction to the divorce. It felt like my life had ended and I was bitterly jealous of the fact that Barbara started dating a younger man. I had to compete with a 28-year-old who had no arthritis. Barbara would be quoted saying they had gone for long walks on the beach, something I couldn't do. I lost my confidence and my will to live. Often I considered suicide. More than once I was seriously concerned about my emotional wellbeing.'[4]

Chris Barnard's emotional wellbeing was so affected that he took one of his strangest decisions yet: he decided to exact revenge on the two women whom he believed had cost him his marriage and his happiness.

'After some days I devised my strategy. The helpers who had spread the unholy rumours had to be punished. I could have murdered the two liars but even in my own confused pathological condition, I was never a violent person. So the answer was a witch-doctor.'[5]

As a South African and a medical specialist to boot, Barnard was thoroughly aware of the supernatural abilities that traditional witch-doctors (sangomas) were rumoured to have. They were considered to have the ability to 'put a curse on people that could cause their victims unbearable suffering'.

'I had also heard that a witch-doctor doesn't have to know his target; all he needs is something that used to belong to the victim. I began searching for a sangoma.'

It turned out to be more difficult than Barnard had imagined.

'Where do you get a man or woman like that to do your dirty work for you?'

Eventually a contact of Barnard's indicated that he knew how to get in touch with a sangoma. A meeting was duly arranged in the thick scrub close to Cape Town's airport. All the witch-doctor wanted was a bottle of gin.

'I thought it was probably needed so he could concoct a mixture that the two women would drink.'

Barnard was greatly disappointment at the meeting with the alleged sangoma. 'He was normal, not at all the terrible being that is often associated with sangomas.

'He assured me he was a sangoma and that he could call on the evil spirits at any time. I explained my situation and asked for the worst punishment he could muster to come down on the two women. Then I handed him the bottle of gin and R500 to speed up the process.'[6]

A few weeks later Barnard ran into the two women in question. Nothing seemed to have happened to them. He told them about what he'd done and they both laughed at him.

'A month later they were still very healthy. All my visit to the sangoma had achieved was making a man drunk on a bottle of gin and with a R500 cash bonus as a sweetener to the deal.'

Barnard's behaviour during this period was a major source of embarrassment in later years.

'When I think back on the months following my divorce, I am ashamed at my despicable behaviour. A man's ego is a complex thing.'

Later Chris would admit that Barbara had been correct to divorce him. 'At the end, it was a marriage that had been wrecked and things were made worse by my arthritis.'[7]

Chris was increasingly losing his will to work as a surgeon. The passion for the work was dimming and his physical condition didn't help matters at all.

His saving grace was his friendship with a Roman Catholic priest, Father Tom Nicholson, who helped Barnard get through this dip in his life.

'When the great healer's heart was broken, he came to me for help. It took a while, but time, courage and the acceptance that there were things that we cannot change, was eventually the cure,' Father Tom said later.[8]

Retirement

A year later, in December 1983, Chris Barnard retired at the early age of 61 years. His arthritis played a big part in his decision.

'Pain has been my constant companion every day and night since I was a student in Minneapolis. To be great at your profession you need to get up in the morning, hungry to go to work. By 1983, when I was ready to retire, the pain had stolen that hunger from me. Rather than operating, I was thinking up excuses to avoid surgery.'[9]

This was not totally unexpected. In a 1978 interview, he had predicted that arthritis was going to affect his career.[10]

'It's simply [at times] impossible to operate as a result of the pain in my hands.'

Rheumatoid arthritis is characterised not only by painful and swollen joints and inflammation, but also tiredness, depression and grumpiness.[11]

Over the years Barnard had received hundreds of home remedies and tons of advice from people all over the world, who had wanted to reach out and help him with his affliction.

'Some of the concoctions were so evil I was too afraid to try them in case they might poison me.'

The problem with the disease is that there are periods of remission so people often think that their specific medicine is a cure, when in fact it may have been used at a time when the disease was going into remission.

It was as if the world wanted to cure Chris Barnard the heart healer.

'I collected these concoctions in an arthritis album. At one time, there were more than 800 cures. Some said put copper pennies behind my right ankle. Another suggested shock treatment. Others suggested green tomato juice, dried pawpaw pips, khaki-bush leaves and soaking [my] hands in brake fluid. One person swore by dog pellets. I couldn't help but wonder about all the old dogs struggling across the beaches on arthritic legs.'[12]

Barnard never made fun of the offerings of help and advice. He believed they were sent with love, but nothing would work.

'There's no cure. There are just natural remissions from time to time.'[13]

Chris was the only Barnard son to be afflicted with the disease.

'I kept asking: "Lord why did I have to get arthritis? If I'm being punished, for what am I being punished?"'[14]

Two situations helped him lift his head and keep going. The first was a close friend who died of cancer. 'Even at the end, he was begging the doctors to do what they could to keep him alive. He felt he still had so much left to do. I realised that with or without arthritis, there was still a lot I could get out of life.'

The second situation was when he watched a young child at the Red Cross Children's Hospital. The child had swallowed caustic soda and burnt his throat.

'The result was he couldn't swallow. So the food he chewed had to be diverted with a tube to a plastic bag he had to carry around. A terrible condition. Nevertheless, he would spend each lunch with the other children, chewing happily while the food fell into the bag. When lunch was over, he went to a small side room where the bag was emptied and the staff fed him with a tube into his stomach. The boy wanted to be as normal as possible and communicate and be with his friends despite his problem. From that day forward I started to concentrate less on what I had lost and more on what I had left.'[15]

Barnard concluded 25 colourful years of service when he retired from Groote Schuur. He playfully suggested that he was expecting a Rolex wristwatch. Instead, the hospital gave him a tie with cleaning instructions that stated it was machine washable.[16]

On his retirement, Barnard said that he couldn't help but be taken back to the memories of his youth when he was a 16-year-old kid who had to leave the dance early.

At the time of his retirement, the field of cardiac surgery was one of the great success stories of medicine.

'It felt like I was leaving a child, a child who had grown and got more sophisticated and bigger than I had ever been able to imagine that day when I put the first heart-lung machine together in the hospital.

'I was glad to have been there to provide my two cents' worth. But it was difficult to leave while the music was still playing.'[17]

Later Barnard would explain that retirement felt like being invited to a lunch and showing up just in time for dinner.

'It was difficult to believe that while I had been so busy with other things, the years had gone by.'[18]

Tragedy

For years Barnard had been a civil servant but after his retirement, he could throw off the shackles of bureaucracy and start making some money. He had bought a large farm in the Karoo and dabbled in the restaurant industry in Cape Town, while continuing to write more books. He was still much in demand on the global speaking circuit where he provided brilliant lectures on hearts and medicine and, later, aging. He was particularly popular on luxury cruise ships where he was often seen in the company of beautiful young women.

While Barnard was in Singapore, he got the news that his eldest son had died.[19]

On 1 March 1984, newspapers around the world ran the story about the death of André Barnard, aged 32. André, known as Boetie, was

Chris's eldest son with Louwtjie. He had been discovered dead in the bathtub and a syringe had been found close by on the floor.[20]

Media speculation was rife that he had committed suicide. Some reports quoted anonymous sources saying that André had been suffering from depression.[21]

Andre Barnard was a paediatrician in private practice, having graduated from UCT in 1975. He was the only Barnard child to become a doctor.

André's wife Gail had arrived home at 7.00am from her night shift at Groote Schuur, where she worked as a nurse, and discovered the doors were locked. She peeked through the windows and saw their two young children still asleep and her husband in the bath. She called the police, who broke down the door.[22]

André's death was a huge blow to both Louwtjie and Chris. At the funeral, which brought the two into contact again after a long time, they consoled each other.

Chris had last seen André alive a few weeks earlier when the family had visited Chris on his farm in the Karoo. 'His smile is all I can remember. He always had a smile, even for the bad guys.

'They said I could go and see my son to say goodbye. I didn't go. I never saw my son dead. I wanted to remember him the way he was, alive and warm and smiling. The person I knew didn't deserve a place in a coffin,' Chris wrote later.[23]

The media turned André's death into another scandal, to the shock and horror of the family.

'People in the public eye are public assets and you cannot expect privacy,' a friend consoled Barnard.

Barnard wrote, 'Even before the body was cold there was more speculation. It kept going for days, with each newspaper driving their own angles. At the funeral, newspapermen pointed long lenses into private moments of grief. The most damage was caused by an unlovely soul who went to scratch around in old newspaper archives and discovered an old, long-forgotten disagreement between me and my dead son and then wrote this into the funeral story.'[24]

Bob Molloy from *The Argus* newspaper also felt that the media had played a bad role in the coverage of André Barnard's death.

'Chris had always been a media target but the coverage of his son's death was disgusting. One journalist found a letter that André wrote as a 15-year-old boy which the journalist used to hit Chris with.'[25]

In this letter, the young André was flailing out in pain and anger at his parents' divorce and he was critical of his father. While Chris and Louwtjie grieved for their dead son, the media once again dragged Chris over the coals for long-forgiven sins.[26]

A post-mortem declared André's death to be an accident. The report stated that André had drowned in the bath as a result of an acute reaction to pain medicine he had injected. He had been taking the medicine to treat the injuries he had sustained in a serious car accident.[27]

Cyclosporine

In addition to his continued lecturing across the globe, Barnard accepted a part-time position as an adviser at the Baptist Medical Center in Oklahoma City. This centre was developing a world-class cardiac programme from the ground up and Barnard spent the next two years providing invaluable assistance.[28]

Elsewhere in America, other specialists, including Shumway and Starzl, were still researching organ transplantation and focusing on trying to resolve the rejection problem. They were helped by the discovery of a drug called cyclosporine in 1971, which would prove to be very effective in combatting rejection.

Cyclosporine was isolated from a fungus growing in Norway. Years of development and research followed, until the American Federal Drug Administration finally approved it for use in 1983.[29]

At Stanford, scientists had also developed a unique biopsy technique that made it easier and quicker to determine if a body was rejecting an organ. Gradually the survival rates for transplant patients began to rise.[30]

By January 1985, a total of 2 465 heart transplants had been performed globally. A four-year survival rate of 42% had been achieved using conventional immune-suppression methods. However, the implementation of cyclosporine was a quantum leap forward and one-year survival rates jumped to an 80%, while five-year survival rates jumped to 71%.[31] Today patients live on average for 25 years with transplanted hearts.

Scandal

The greatest scandal in Barnard's later life started out as a friendship with Armin Mattli, the owner of a Swiss health clinic that was well known for helping the who's who of the rich and famous to recapture their beauty and youthful vitality.[32]

In the 1980s, manufacturers of skin products started to emphasise their breakthrough research relating to the repair of cellular tissue.[33]

In 1985, Mattli contracted Barnard to become the spokesperson and face of his company's new skin cream, a product called Glycel. This was marketed as a product for eternal youth that could 'heal wounds, remove wrinkles and make skin look younger for longer'[34]

The marketing material claimed that the chief ingredient, glycosphingolipid, had been tested on damaged cells and proved to have regenerative properties that could 'make older skin look younger'.[35] This research was not published. It also stated that the great scientist Barnard had worked on the development of the product, together with a team of researchers at the Schaefer Institute in Switzerland.[36]

Glycel was distributed by a company called Alfin Fragrances at a cost of between US$25 and US$75. And these were small pots.[37]

Barnard's decision to get involved with Glycel paid off financially but did his reputation enormous damage, particularly in medical circles.

On 16 April 1986, the *Chicago Tribune* wrote about its surprise at discovering that Barnard was playing a leading role in the marketing of Glycel, described as being a skin cream that promised to delay the aging process. According to the paper, Barnard, 63 years old, described his latest project as being 'just another aspect of my medical career'.

'I'm [still] trying to improve the quality of life of people. I think one can improve the quality of people's lives significantly by finding out all one can about the aging process. What is wrong with that?'[38]

He was accused of doing this for the money.

'I'm retired and my pension is US$400 per month. I need an additional income.'[39]

Some sources claimed that Barnard had been paid US$4 million to have his name attached to Glycel. Barnard, however, denied this and claimed he'd never been paid more than US$200 000.[40]

He was slammed for not being a dermatologist, yet lending his face and reputation to a skin product.

Dr Norman Orentreich, a well-known Manhattan dermatologist, described Barnard as a 'huckster medical man'.[41] Orentreich, who had done 40 years of research in the field, stated that the claims that Glycel was making could not be substantiated.

Irwin Alfin, the owner of Alfin Fragrances, reacted by saying that critics of Glycel were being negative because they were working for competing cosmetics companies.[42] He also made it clear that his company had made no medical claims about the products and said that the results of the scientific research into the product had not been published because of the highly competitive nature of the cosmetics business.

'We are not in the academic sciences or the medical field. No-one in our industry publishes [research] and therefore we won't do it either.[43]

Glycel was eventually withdrawn from the American market in 1987 because of unrelenting pressure and later Barnard admitted that punting Glycel was his greatest regret.

'It was the single greatest error I made in my life.'

In an article published in *New York Magazine* in November 1985, which discussed Barnard's involvement with Glycel, there's a photo of Barnard with a young woman standing behind him. The caption reads

'Christiaan Barnard with a friend'.[44]

The friend was Karin Setzkorn. Three years later she would become the third Mrs Barnard.

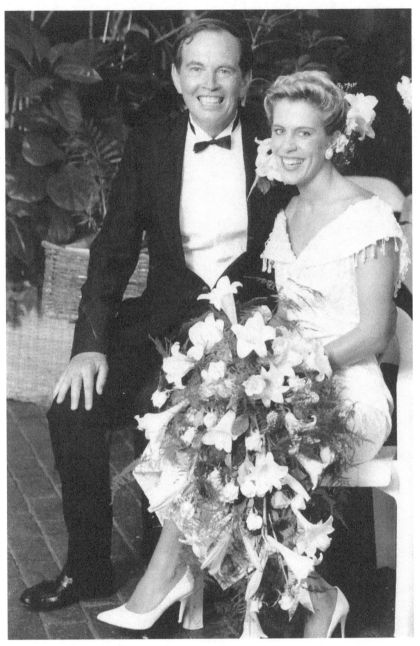

In 1988 Christiaan Barnard got married to Karin Setzkorn in Cape Town.

CHAPTER 17

Full circle

O N SATURDAY, 23 JANUARY 1988, 65-YEAR-OLD CHRISTIAAN BAR-
nard got married for the third time, this time to Karin Setzkorn, a
24-year-old model.[1]

Chris had met her a few years earlier when she was 19 and working
as a waitress in Cape Town. Chris and Karin got married in a 15-min-
ute civil ceremony, followed by a party held at a restaurant Chris had
bought in Cape Town. The couple had wanted to get married in Father
Tom's Roman Catholic Church, but the church would not condone the
marriage as Chris was a divorced man. There were 130 guests, including
several top surgeons from across the globe.[2]

A huge media scrum erupted over the wedding, mainly between the
Sunday papers. *Rapport* newspaper had bought the exclusive rights for
the event but its competitor, the *Sunday Times*, had found a photograph
of Karin as a young girl sitting on Barnard's lap. It was obviously an old
photograph taken when the two coincidentally met during a holiday a
long time before.[3]

The VIP guests included Chris's boss from Oklahoma City, Dr Nazih
Zuhdi, and his wife. Zuhdi recalled later that the ceremony was held in
the parsonage next to the church.[4]

'The priest was a loyal friend of Chris's. The reception was held at
the restaurant called La Vita. The police on horseback had to keep the
crowd away.'

Zuhdi and his wife accompanied the Barnards on the first part of their
honeymoon, a trip to Johannesburg on the famous Blue Train.

'When the train stopped in Beaufort West for 30 minutes there were hundreds of people [from the coloured community] on the platform to welcome Chris and Karin. They were there singing and dancing. Chris had always remained their hero because he had always stood up for the oppressed and less privileged.'[5]

From Johannesburg, the Barnards went to MalaMala, an exclusive game reserve.

For the next few years, the Barnards were less in the news and Chris started to focus on his 32 000-acre sheep and game farm in the Karoo, close to Richmond.[6] He also kept writing and completed his fourth novel, *The Donor*, which was published in 1996.

The international speaking circuit was still a haven but his talks now included controversial topics such as euthanasia, which he endorsed.

'I'm not in favour of active euthanasia, but certainly for passive. All doctors practise a measure of passive euthanasia. At times, it is simply better for a patient in terms of alleviating suffering, to stop further treatment.'

Lady Diana

If there was one person who knew what Chris Barnard had been through when it came to the media, it was Lady Diana. It seems that destiny brought the two together and they became friends.[7]

The two often met at Kensington Palace in London, where Diana was staying after her separation from Prince Charles in 1992. The basis for their friendship was the idea of creating a heart foundation for children. Diana wanted Chris to continue with the work he'd been doing as a surgeon – saving the lives of children with serious heart conditions. As a surgeon, Chris had done pro bono heart surgery on hundreds of poor children, many from developing countries, whose families had no means of paying for the procedures. This work done by Barnard has been largely forgotten by many of his critics.

'Chris would spend days beside the beds of these desperately ill children tending to them personally. I often found he was operating three days per week at Red Cross Children's Hospital, where he would operate during the day, spend the night next to the child's bed and repeat this again for another two days straight. That attention was very often the difference between life and death for those children,' says Otto Thaning.[8]

Since his arthritis had made it impossible for Barnard to continue doing the procedures personally, a new solution had to be found. Barnard also knew money was needed and this was where Diana could have had a huge impact as a patron. Their relationship grew from discussions relating to the foundation, and the plans were on course until Diana's untimely and tragic death on 31 August 1997 in a car accident in Paris.

Barnard remained determined to keep Diana's dream alive and with the support of the Arthur Andersen Group in 1998 he established the Christiaan Barnard Foundation. For some years this foundation did remarkable work, and many of the operations were performed by a new top South African heart surgeon, one of the world's few female heart surgeons and a good friend of Barnard's, Dr Susan Vosloo. (The 10-year-old Sheri, who had wanted to know if women could also be heart surgeons, would have been proud to hear this!)

Barnard's friendship with Diana has another interesting twist and this relates to another dream Diana had – the dream to make a new life for herself in South Africa.

Diana's death has linked her for all time to a playboy named Dodi Al-Fayed, who died in the same car crash.[9] For years, however, the rumour has been circulating that Diana's relationship with Al-Fayed had been little more than a flirtation aimed at winning back the affection of a man who had broken up with her. This man was a Pakistani heart surgeon named Hasnat Khan.

Diana met Khan on 1 September 1995. Her relationship with Khan was kept a secret for a long time, but the two dated for around two years, spending time in Kensington Palace where they could avoid the paparazzi.[10]

Khan was a serious man who often spent 90-hour weeks working as a surgeon in the National Health Service in England. The two of them discussed marriage and Diana even introduced him to her two sons. But Khan remained wary of all the media attention Diana was still getting.

In July 1996, Charles offered Diana a divorce.

Sally Bedell Smith's book, *Diana in Search of Herself: Portrait of a Troubled Princess*, claims that Diana was madly in love with Khan and prepared to convert to Islam if that was what it would take to marry the heart surgeon.[11]

In October 1996, Diana went to Italy where she received a humanitarian award together with Barnard. On this occasion, she asked Barnard if he could arrange a job for Khan as a heart surgeon in South Africa.[12]

'Diana begged Dr Barnard to get him [Khan] work in South Africa. She wanted to have daughters with him and was thinking of putting up a home close to her brother.'[13]

Diana's brother, Earl Spencer, was living in the Cape Town suburb of Constantia at the time.

Barnard said that he would see what he could do. Sadly, this didn't work out, despite Barnard's best efforts. The problem was probably because Barnard had very little influence left in Cape Town circles, especially at state-run institutions like Groote Schuur Hospital.

'The head of Groote Schuur's Cardiothoracic Department in the late 1990s also had little respect for Prof Barnard. Seemingly he couldn't understand the advantages it could have held [had Khan been appointed] for the department,' says Vosloo, who was still working in the department at the time.

For Diana, a story that could have had a happy ending, ended tragically. First Khan left her – largely due to the insane media attention she was getting – and then she died in a car accident in a dark Parisian tunnel, surrounded by paparazzi.

Khan still lives in England where he continues to work as a cardiac surgeon.[14]

Barbara dies

Another tragedy struck in 1998, when Barbara died of breast cancer at the age of 48. She had remarried, to Joe da Silva, with whom she had a daughter.

Barbara's mother, Ulli, had died in 1995, also from breast cancer. Ulli's death was traumatic and Chris had to step in at the end and suggest that the machines keeping her alive be switched off to prevent her prolonged suffering.

Fred Zoellner, Barbara's billionaire father, died of a heart attack only days before his daughter and left his huge fortune to Barbara. But three days later she, too, died.

Barbara's death hit Chris hard and he was inconsolable at the funeral. Time and old age were finally catching up with the pioneering surgeon and his health started to deteriorate rapidly, as had his third marriage to Karin. The age difference between Karin and Chris made things difficult and they, too, started drifting apart. It didn't help matters when Karin discovered Viagra in Chris's valise.[15] (Chris, however, always insisted that he never used Viagra.)[16] By this time, the couple were no longer sharing a bedroom.

The Telegraph, a British tabloid, reported that Karin was divorcing Chris after his 'Viagra-fuelled affair with a younger woman'.

The old playboy had stepped into his final pothole and his third divorce was finalised in March 2000. Karin was 35 years old. The two had been married for 11 years and they had two small children, Armin and Lara.

Full circle

The last years of Chris Barnard's life were in some ways often lonely and difficult. He established himself partly in Vienna, Austria, where the Christiaan Barnard Foundation had headquarters, and partly in Cape Town, where his family was.

In Cape Town, Barnard made his new home in an apartment in Oranjezicht. However, he considered Austria to be a more peaceful environment and said that he wanted to escape the emotional and physical pain that was in South Africa. His partner in the Christiaan Barnard Foundation, Walter Lutschinger, was also based Vienna. Barnard was seeking a new start in a city that still treated him like a hero.[17]

By this time, he was struggling with his health and then he was diagnosed with a melanoma on his nose. A part of his nose had to be cut away and skin grafts were made using skin from his forehead. This was a hammer blow for a man who had been known across the world as a playboy and whose youthful good looks had meant so much to him. He joked about the operation and said that he had actually received a facelift.

'Now I need to shave behind my ears,' he joked.[18]

But there is no doubt that the loss of his looks was a bitter blow. Barnard had changed from being one of the world's most desirable people to one who was almost unacceptable to himself. Matters only got worse when he stumbled over a step in Vienna and broke his hip.[19]

In South Africa, he went for a hip replacement and acknowledged for the first time that he was 'feeling like an old man'.

But the old Barnard was still there. In his last book, *50 Ways to a Healthy Heart*, published in 2001, Barnard writes that 'nothing keeps a heart healthier than regular sex'.[20]

Barnard's life came full circle towards the end, when he and Louwtjie became friendly again. This was largely thanks to Deirdre, their eldest daughter, who was the bridge between her parents. In Cape Town, Chris lived a little way up towards Table Mountain from Deirdre, and Louwtjie not far below her. Deirdre would sometimes go for a gin and tonic with her dad or a whisky with her mum. But often the three of them would simply meet up at Deirdre's home. Louwtjie started tailoring Chris's clothes again, often shortening his trousers. Like old times, she also started cooking offal for her old partner.

'Chris loved offal and it was the one thing Louwtjie could really do well. So she made Chris offal again,' recalls Andre Wagner, a family member.

'At the end, Chris was very vulnerable and he returned to the place he felt safe – with Louwtjie and Deirdre.'

The three Barnards would visit one another regularly and reminisce, although Louwtjie, on occasion, still hauled Chris over the coals in her straight-shooting manner.[21]

In those final years, Wagner often drove Chris around the city.

'He often said that at the end of one's life, the only question that really matters is, "Have you made a difference?"'

Death

In 1980 Chris Barnard wrote about death as follows: 'Everyone must die. You reading these words and I writing them. Death is the only certainty of life, no matter if it comes sooner or later, gradually or suddenly. It is a situation which we should all bear in mind and in our mortality, we are all equal.'[22]

Twenty-one years later, on 2 September 2001, Chris Barnard's heart beat for the last time. He was 78 years old and visiting a resort in Paphos, a city on the southwest coast of the Mediterranean island of Cyprus.[23] Barnard was a regular visitor to Paphos, where he had been given the freedom of the city earlier that year.[24]

This visit was not for pleasure only; he was finalising a new business venture, marketing olive oil. After Paphos he was scheduled to visit Germany, where he was going to meet with the country's largest meat distributor.

'He wanted to negotiate distributing springbok meat from his farm in the Karoo in Germany. Springbok meat has no cholesterol and the Germans were very excited at the prospects,' Lutschinger told *Huisgenoot* after Barnard's death.[25]

The evening before Chris died, he attended a dinner and appeared to enjoy himself with the other guests. The following morning, he suffered a fatal asthma attack and died beside the Coral Beach Hotel's swimming pool.[26]

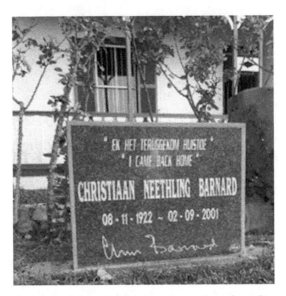

*'I came back home'. Christiaan Barnard was buried in
the family's old garden in Beaufort-West.*

© AMANDA HUGHES

By this time he had been suffering from asthma for a while and he had
forgotten his asthma inhaler in his room. A load of chlorine had just
been added to the pool and breathing in the chlorine fumes may have set
off the asthma attack.

At the time of his death, the world view on heart transplants had
progressed significantly since the early days of Washkansky. The development of the powerful anti-rejection drugs had made heart transplants
a standard procedure.[27]

By 2001, the estimated number of heart transplants stood at 100 000
worldwide. In January 1985, there had been only 2 465. This dramatic
increase shows the massive impact that the new drugs had had. *The New
York Times* reported that at the time of Barnard's death, heart transplants
were being performed in 160 hospitals across America alone. The one-year
survival rate had shot up to 90% and the five-year survival rate to 75%.[28]

It was a long way from the poor results in the 1960s when the majority of patients were dying and heart-transplant centres were all being shut down, barring four, including Groote Schuur.

Curiously, at the end, it was not the heart transplant that Chris wished to be remembered for.

'If I had to be remembered one day, I would like to be remembered for the work I did with children. I consider that to be my greatest success.'

The world reacts

In the 21 years since Marius Barnard had left Groote Schuur, he had seen his brother very seldom due in part to Chris's new family commitments and Marius's new career path. Chris's death came as a shock to his younger brother. Marius was fighting cancer and had always believed he would be dead before Chris. In his memoirs, Marius expresses regret that they didn't see more of one another. Marius and Inéz, his wife of nearly 50 years, were in Namaqualand for the flower season, the weekend Chris died.[29]

'Late on the Sunday afternoon, close to Cape Town, I switched my cellphone back on. Voice messages. The first was from an ex-colleague who sympathised with the death of my brother. I phoned Louwtjie and Deirdre answered. She confirmed that her dad had died that day.

'I was shocked. The one who was meant to die was me. I had been struggling with cancer for 13 years already,' Marius recounts.

Vicky Georges was a pianist at the Coral Beach Hotel. After Barnard's death, she wrote a long letter to Chris's youngest daughter, the four-year-old Lara, in which she told Lara about her father's last evening.

'He came to the piano, introduced himself, kissed my hand and asked that I play "Lara's Theme" from Dr Zhivago for him. He said it was for his daughter, Lara. "She's in Africa … my family is there."'

On the day of Chris Barnard's death, Louwtjie was with Deirdre when the media started calling. Deirdre asked her mother what she should say about her father.

'Tell them he was a wonderful man, he made wonderful medical advancements – and he was full of monkey business.'

Nelson Mandela was one of thousands who sympathised with the Barnards. 'I admired him a lot and I'm sorry that he has left us.'[30]

Barnard was survived by five of his six children, Deirdre, Christiaan, Frederick, Armin and Lara, one adopted son, André, two ex-wives, Louwtjie and Karin, and his brother Marius. The heart pioneer had four memorial services, two in Cape Town and two in Beaufort West.

Some years earlier, Chris had buried the hatchet with his old home-town and the town turned his father's old church and the old parsonage into a museum, which can still be visited today. Christiaan Barnard, the man who had been as far away as one could be from the troubled little Karoo town, a man who had had the world at his feet, was buried in the garden of the old parsonage in which he was born.

The headstone simply reads, 'I came back home'.

CHAPTER 18

Legacy

3 December 2016

T HE MAJESTIC NEW CHRISTIAAN BARNARD MEMORIAL HOSPITAL IN
Cape Town's city bowl is complete. It's 50 years since the passing of
Chris Barnard and people's memories are fading. Most people remember three things about Chris Barnard when asked. He transplanted the
first human heart successfully, he hailed from Beaufort West and he was
very fond of women. One person suggested that the sentence construc-
tion should read, 'he was fond of many women'.

After his death, there was much controversy to which his name was
connected. The Hamilton Naki matter was discussed. There was also a
false allegation that the Barnard brothers had stopped Denise Darvall's
heart with potassium and did not wait for it to stop beating on its own.
In 2003, a British tabloid, *The Telegraph*, accused Barnard of wanting
to remove Darvall's heart while she was still alive.[1] But Denise Darvall's
stopped of its own accord.

Following Washkansky's transplant, and for years thereafter, a bitter
war of words was exchanged, especially from American and British medical circles, accusing Chris Barnard of stealing Shumway's and Lower's
research and acting unethically to beat them to the punch.

The Groote Schuur team's heart-transplant results were unparalleled
in the world and would remain so for decades before the arrival of cyclosporine. Although Louis Washkansky lived for only 18 days with his
second heart, four of Chris's first 10 patients lived for longer than a year.

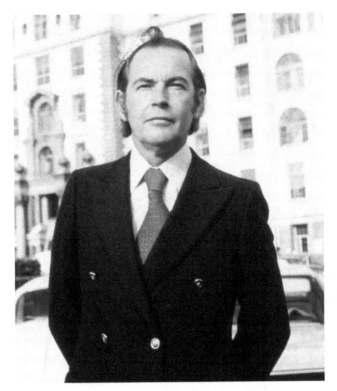

Radical. Outspoken. Courageous. Controversial. Many words
describe Christiaan Barnard, but perhaps 'pioneer' is best.

PHOTOGRAPH COURTESY OF THE HEART OF CAPE TOWN MUSEUM

The Groote Schuur doctors did a great deal more pioneering, including the piggyback heart operations, and later they were the first to transport donor hearts successfully by means of hypothermic storage equipment.[2]

Barnard's work with children at the Red Cross Children's Hospital was world class and the picture of sick children who previously had no hope, leaving with pink cheeks and healthy hearts has been imprinted in the minds of many people.

The Barnard brothers and their team broke every political rule. Their hospital wards were desegregated from the very beginning. Chris Barnard insisted on allowing all nursing staff to tend to white patients, and vice versa, regardless of colour. One American patient on whom Barnard operated, said that he hoped he would receive a white heart. Barnard answered that he wouldn't be able to say since one couldn't tell them apart.[3]

The Barnard brothers set up heart programmes behind the Iron Curtain in communist countries such as Romania, where Marius is still highly esteemed today. They did not hesitate to step on political toes and through it all, stuck to their principles.

All over the world today, the biggest challenge regarding heart transplantation is finding sufficient donors. The next breakthrough may well be artificial hearts and other mechanical devices to keep patients alive until donor hearts become available. Experiments are still being done with animal organs.[4]

Towards the end of his life, Shumway said that he considered Barnard's greatest contribution to be around changing the perceptions around using brain-dead patients as organ donors.

'It was a monumental step forward, because it was applicable for all other organ transplants,' Shumway said.[5]

Politics

There are another one or two anecdotes to be told about Chris Barnard's political views. He himself questioned what patriotism was.

'Is patriotism a sin? My patriotic instinct is compared to racism by television interviewers who decided that I was a monster because I tried to defend my country. What may be necessary is a definition of true patriotism, a problem comparable to true religion. I still haven't fathomed what patriotism is, but I have a vague idea of what it is not.

As Pik Botha said, '"I'm not prepared to die for a sign on the door of a lift. The way I see it, patriots speak to people. Patriots accept the fact that we are all in the same boat. Patriots encourage people to play for the same team. Patriots are colour blind. Without that sort of patriotism in my country, we don't stand a chance in hell"'.[6]

Andre Wagner says that Chris's views and lifestyle proved that he was always patriotic towards South Africa.

'It was important during the 1970s and 1980s to be the type of patriot that is neither a nationalist nor a racist. A prophet is sadly often not recognised in his own country.'[7]

Father Tom Nicholson, who got to know him later in his life, said that Barnard had an unusual sensitivity towards the problems and questions of his time.

'He would often be heartbroken and disappointed because he did so little to change things. It was difficult for him to grasp the suffering in the world, especially the suffering of children and the innocent. He always questioned "How can a God of love allow it?"'[8]

At the time of Barnard's death, President Thabo Mbeki described Barnard as a symbol of excellence and humanity.

'South Africa has lost a great man who made an excellent contribution to his country.'

Fame

After the heart transplant, Chris Barnard experienced more fame than most, before or since. He danced with princesses and visited the Pope. This prominence came at a great personal cost, not least of which were his three marriages.

Nevertheless, Barnard was the first to admit that he enjoyed the attention. 'Anybody that says they do not like being applauded and acknowledged is either a fool or a liar.'[9]

Barnard had a good sense of humour. Once at a sport presentation ceremony in Durban, he jokingly said that someday he would transplant a brain.

'We can, for example, transplant the brain of a doctor into the body of a rugby player. That will be one giant step towards creating the ideal sportsman.'[10]

He concluded that speech on a serious note and cautioned against being a bad loser.

'Don't perform and carry on when you have lost, but don't be satisfied with the result.'[11]

Otto Thaning said that it is human to put heroes on podiums. 'But then the masses come with every effort to dethrone those heroes. It is easier to pull one person down than for everyone else to rise to that level.'

Thaning related a story about a boat that was grounded at low tide among all the other boats in the harbour.

'That boat, same as the others, cannot do much. Then the tide comes in and lifts all those boats. Suddenly there are so many more possibilities. Chris Barnard was that incoming tide.'

In his memoir, published in 2011, Marius Barnard wrote about his brother as follows:

'After his death, attempts were made to keep Chris alive but it got more difficult. People forget. Chris played a tremendous role in the history of heart surgery. He will always be remembered as the first to transplant a heart and so his name will live on. He will, nevertheless, also be remembered for the less pleasant things. His personal life was manna for the relentless media that firstly uplifted him and then with great pleasure tore him down. My brother realised too late the danger of manmade honour.'[12]

Marius says that in the end, Chris's appearance, of which he was so proud and which he tried so hard to protect, was maimed by cancer and surgery.

'In the end, he found love and care again in Louwtjie and Deirdre … The wheel had turned. Full circle.'[13]

Throughout Chris Barnard's life, he received a lot of criticism for his personal life, including his three marriages and numerous love affairs.

Johan Naude, an ex-colleague and fellow-surgeon at Groote Schuur, wrote in his memoir: 'I worked 18-hour days, never a day off and often in 24- to 36-hour stretches. My marriage crumbled and my children and I became estranged.'

Naude said that, as surgeons, the fact that they made life-and-death decisions was never a conscious one and definitely not one that they examined intellectually, but emotionally it took its toll and they could not escape.

'It caused chaos in our lives. We became arrogant and thought our-selves to be above the law and above the morality which manages the rest of humankind. Nobody's marriage lasted over the long haul, with the exception of Marius Barnard.'[14]

One captain

Barnard's breakthroughs levelled the field for a world that was ready for progress. Great medical breakthroughs are the result of the inputs and hard work of various pioneers over a period of many years.

Barnard was a pathfinder and pioneer. Pioneering is not the result of a single individual's efforts. Chris Barnard was fully aware of this and admitted it chivalrously.

Chris's brother Marius, a key role-player and stalwart of the Groote Schuur team, together with the rest of the heart team, including sur-geons such as Hewitson and other specialists like Ozinsky and Schrire, were world-class.

There was, however, one captain.

'In 1997, at the 30th anniversary of the first heart transplant, Barnard gave a party for the original heart team,' remembers Susan Vosloo.

'He was aware of the role that each member filled and acknowledged each one, after which he described them as links in a chain – a chain that was only as strong as its weakest link.'

A large cartoon at the Heart of Cape Town Museum is a poster by the cartoonist TO Honiball depicting the whole heart team. This was done after Chris once mentioned that there was never a proper pho-tograph taken of all the team members together. The cartoon depicts the medical practitioners as baboons, which was Honiball's style, in an orchestra. Facing the orchestra is the conductor. That conductor is Chris Barnard.

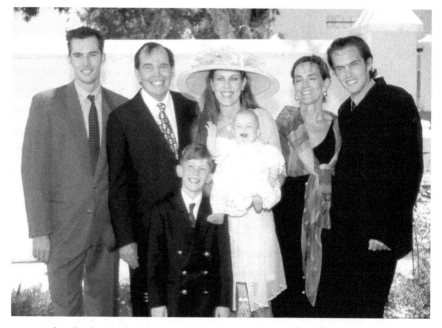

*A family photo of the Barnards taken at Lara Barnard's christening in 1997.
From left to right: Frederick, Chris, Armin (in front), Karin (holding Lara),
Deirdre and Christiaan (jnr).*

PHOTOGRAPH COURTESY OF THE HEART OF CAPE TOWN MUSEUM

Work with children

The Red Cross War Memorial Children's Hospital is the biggest teaching
hospital in South Africa erected exclusively for children. It was erected as
a memorial to the soldiers of all races who sacrificed so much during the
Second World War. Returning ex-soldiers felt that children had suffered
most during the war.

This hospital – with a Peter Pan statue at the entrance – is where Chris
Barnard tended and healed hordes of children for decades. The hospital
today treats around 260 000 patients per year, the overwhelming majority of whom come from underprivileged communities. One-third of all
these patients are younger than one year.

The hospital's proud ethos is that no child will be turned away and the hospital's policy includes open visiting hours to allow parents to be part of their children's healing process.[15]

The Barnard brothers were there for the majority of the great breakthroughs at this hospital, operations that made Red Cross an island on a continent where no other such hospitals existed.

This hospital was responsible for many of the first operations done on children in Africa, such as the first separation of Siamese twins in 1964 and the first kidney transplant on a child in 1968.

The Chris Barnard Department for Heart Surgery

The Chris Barnard Department for Heart Surgery still forms part of UCT's Department of Surgery. This department exclusively treats underprivileged patients with no medical aid. After the advent of democracy in 1994, new priorities resulted in the department losing more than half of its beds in wards and in the intensive care unit. Instead, government budgets were channelled into programmes such as HIV/Aids and tuberculosis. Specialist programmes, such as cardiac surgery, saw a sharp decline in funding from the mid-1990s. It was seen as costly speciality treatment exclusively for individuals who could afford it.

A typical developed-world cardiac centre budgets for 800–1 000 openheart operations per million adults per year. In Cape Town, the two public hospitals performing heart operations are Groote Schuur and Tygerberg. Together these have to take care of six million people, yet only 700 heart operations are performed on adults annually.

In South Africa, the number of heart operations offered to underprivileged communities countrywide is rapidly diminishing. In 1992, the national budget for heart operations allowed for approximately 142 operations per million people. By 2001, this had diminished to 66 per million while the identified need at that time stood at 356 per million.

Taking into consideration population growth since 2001, when Chris Barnard died, it has become apparent that only every 8th to 10th indigent patient needing heart surgery in South Africa can be helped today. The reality, however, is that heart disease, especially among the poorer communities, is rapidly increasing. The World Health Organisation (WHO) warns that by 2020, heart disease will be the number-one killer of people in developing countries.

Groote Schuur heart transplants after Barnard

The Cardiology Division at Groote Schuur Hospital was named after Barnard and sustained an active heart-transplant programme, even after his death, albeit limited.[16]

By the mid-1990s, Groote Schuur Hospital was performing about 30 heart transplants annually, but since then, the largest contingent of patients who can afford a heart transplant have turned to the private sector. By the late 1990s, the division was doing fewer than 10 heart transplants annually.

By 2000, the division was in financial trouble and was on the brink of closing down, when professors Peter Zilla and Johan Brink took over. Brink's efforts to find a new partner led to Netcare, the largest private hospital group in South Africa. This group took co-ownership of the division and since then things have stabilised.

In 1973, transplant programmes were available only in public hospitals, including Johannesburg General and Baragwanath in Johannesburg, HF Verwoerd in Pretoria, Addington in Durban and Groote Schuur in Cape Town. By 1982, Universitas in Bloemfontein and Tygerberg in Cape Town also started with transplantation. Today there are 18 transplant centres in South Africa, 8 government and 10 private facilities.[17]

There are still approximately 4 300 South Africans at any one time waiting for organ donations. In 2015, there were 548 organ and corneal transplants in South Africa. This included 27 adult hearts.[18]

Despite challenges, there is still world-class research on the go at UCT's Cardiology Division. A flagship project at the moment is the development of a new type of artificial heart valve under the auspices of professors Peter Zilla, David Williams and Deon Bezuidenhout. The work is being done in conjunction with a company named Strait Access Technologies. The research involves developing an affordable solution for use in developing countries where rheumatic heart disease affects approximately 75 million people annually. Heather Coombes, one of the leaders of the project, says that the team hopes to introduce the new product to the market by 2018.

'The idea is to produce a heart valve that can be implanted into the heart without open-heart surgery. It will impact tremendously as costs and additional treatment will be eliminated.'

The Nobel Prize controversy

One of the biggest disappointments in Chris Barnard's life was the fact that he never won the Nobel Prize. On 17 April 1968, the Brazilian medical profession nominated Barnard for the 1968 Nobel Prize in Physiology or Medicine.[19]

He did not receive the prize, however, and on 4 October 1968, the Nobel Institute announced that the award had been given to three American scientists, Robert Holley, Har Gobind Khorana and Marshall Nirenberg, for their research on how genes control human cells.[20]

Barnard caused a controversy when in an interview in 1997 with *Frontline*, an Indian magazine, he speculated that he had not won the Nobel Prize because a white South African at the time would have been an unpopular choice.

Interestingly, the Nobel Institute has a rule that it does not answer questions about candidates until 50 years after the award ceremony. Accordingly, it offered only some guidance on queries about Chris Barnard and the 1968 award.

'Please contact the Nobel offices in 2019 and we will answer your questions regarding the 1968 nominations. Till that time, we will only broadly supply information concerning the rules of the Nobel Prize. We cannot concentrate specifically on the individual in question,' stated Ann-Mari Dumanski, the Nobel officer who deals with

Physiology or Medicine. Dumanski explained that the Nobel Prize is allocated to the person that has made the most important discovery in the domain of Physiology or Medicine, as stated in Alfred Nobel's testament.

'For example, lifelong achievements, capable researchers or doctors are not what Alfred Nobel had in mind; he specifically mentioned discovery.'

It would be interesting to see in 2019 if any researchers were invited to judge the adequacy of awarding the prize to Chris Barnard. If that were the case, the only qualified candidates would have been American and the majority of them did not favour Chris Barnard. In 1968, they still felt that he had unfairly jumped the gun on their fellow Americans, Lower and Shumway. Most researchers were unaware of the research done by the Barnard brothers over almost 10 years prior to the heart transplant.

'All archive material remains a secret for 50 years, after which it can possibly be given to researchers to investigate. Nationality, sex and the rest is of no importance to the Nobel committee in Physiology or Medicine. Alfred Nobel stated clearly that his wish was that the award of the prizes would give no consideration to the nationality of the candidates, but that the most worthy will receive the prize,' Dumanski said on behalf of the institution.

Barnard commented once that if he had to choose between the Nobel Prize and a pretty woman, he would choose the latter.[21]

Deirdre says her father was kidding. 'He would have really wanted the Nobel Prize.'

Given that the award in this category is usually awarded to more than one person, why wasn't it awarded to Barnard, Shumway and Lower? Unless there were other reasons that disqualified Chris. Shumway and Lower could not have won the prize without Barnard being included. This must have been a heavy blow to the Americans and could have cost Chris Barnard too.

We will wait and see in 2019.

A bag of tools
RL Sharpe

Isn't it strange
That princes and kings,
And clowns that caper
In sawdust rings,
And common people
Like you and me
Are builders for eternity?

Each is given a bag of tools,
A shapeless mass,
A book of rules;
And each must make —
Ere life is flown —
A stumbling block
Or a steppingstone.

This was one of Christiaan Barnard's favourite poems, read by Frederick at his father's funeral.

Epilogue

IN SOUTH AFRICA, 210 PEOPLE DIE EVERY DAY OF HEART-RELATED DISEASE.[1] No-one is immune to heart-related diseases but some are more vulnerable than others, namely children and the poor. They are particularly susceptible to contracting rheumatic fever, which can destroy their hearts, as was the case with Dorothy Fischer. The impact of rheumatic heart disease is set to increase rapidly and cause many more fatalities among poorer populations in developing countries.[2]

In South Africa, heart disease is the leading cause of death among children under the age of 5. The WHO says that heart disease has become the leading cause of death across the globe today.

In 2015 approximately 17.7 million people died of heart disease, roughly 31% of all deaths recorded that year. Of the 17.7 million, about 7.4 million people died from coronary heart failure and 6.7 million died from strokes. More than three-quarters of these deaths occurred in low- and middle-income areas – countries like South Africa.[3]

Deaths due to heart disease in sub-Saharan Africa are predicted to increase dramatically into the future due to the upsurge in urbanisation. Lifestyle choices, including less exercise and poor dietary choices, as well as high blood pressure will have an increasing impact on people in developing countries like South Africa.[4]

The work done by hospitals like Groote Schuur and the breakthroughs made in Cape Town therefore cannot be underemphasised.

The big question is whether the important work being done on heart disease at state-funded hospitals will get the proper acknowledgement it deserves and the resultant support it requires, especially in terms of funding for research and treatment. In the future, there is no doubt that these medical institutions will come under increased pressure due to the increasing number of people, especially from poorer areas, who will be contracting heart disease.

Huge choices lie ahead for African governments if they want to have any impact on the situation in future.

Fifty years

December 2017 is the 50th anniversary of the first heart transplant done in Theatre A.

Christiaan Barnard has been dead for 16 years. His brother Marius died in 2014. The bulk of the team have passed on too.

The people who remember those heady days are growing fewer and fewer as the years pass. Pik Botha says there are few South Africans who are historically irreplaceable and irrefutable.

'Chris Barnard's achievements paid no heed to race or status. They were for the benefit of people, all people. Across the world. At the end of it all, we're all just people on Earth. And at the end, it just depends on what your contribution was towards a better world.'

In 1982, it was the 15th anniversary of the first heart transplant at Groote Schuur. Chris reassessed the operation that had changed so many lives in one of his *Cape Times* columns.[5]

'One commentator said that while top surgeons worldwide were ready to do the operation, it was pure luck that the first one happened in South Africa. I agree, wholeheartedly. It was luck to be born to parents for whom second best wasn't good enough. It was luck that my application for medicine was accepted at an institution of UCT's calibre.

'Years later it was luck that I was accepted by UCT to be trained as a surgeon. And it was a fluke that made me walk across campus one day and bump into the head of a department that told me about an opening in Minneapolis that offered exciting research possibilities.

'The luck just kept coming.

'I finished my internal medicine and went to Minneapolis where I was offered an apprenticeship in general surgery. When that was done, they offered me a position in Cardiology.

'My luck held.

'I was accepted as an assistant on a heart team.

'I felt I couldn't expect more luck, until I arrived back in Cape Town, and found that the calibre of people manning the hospital were among the best the world had to offer. With that type of luck, could the heart transplant have happened anywhere else?'

In 2011 Cape Town renamed a number of streets that had apartheid-era names. The process was put into motion when the Eastern Boulevard freeway, which brings travellers into the city, was renamed Nelson Mandela Boulevard in honour of the ex-president and freedom fighter. The Mandela name change was done three days before the icon's 93rd birthday on 18 July 2011.

Several months later, on 8 November 2011, the Western Boulevard into the city was renamed Helen Suzman Boulevard, in honour of the anti-apartheid politician. On 3 December 2011, more name changes were made, including Modderdam Road being renamed Robert Sobukwe Road.

And in the foreshore area, close to the harbour, Oswald Pirow Street was renamed Christiaan Barnard Street. During the ceremony, the Mayor of Cape Town, Patricia de Lille, described Barnard as 'one of Cape Town's greatest sons'.

'We honour the best of our city through giving recognition to the pioneer of one of the twentieth century's biggest triumphs.'

The mayor was referring back to a Sunday morning on 3 December 1967, when Dr Christiaan Barnard led a team of 30 South Africans in an epic medical operation that shook the world – the first successful heart transplant.

Acknowledgements

A project like this would have been impossible without the work done by those writers who have gone before. There are many books about Chris Barnard and the first heart transplant, many of which were written by the surgeon himself. There are also many volumes of newsprint and online sources, including medical journals, university and museum archives, and other authoritative archives, that contain information on what was accomplished in Cape Town in 1967 and beyond.

I am most thankful for the work that went before, work that helped guide this book, sometimes in strange directions. A book that was invaluable was one edited and compiled by David Cooper titled *Chris Barnard: By Those Who Know Him*. It contains many interviews and comments by Barnard's friends, family and colleagues, most of whom are no longer around. Chris Barnard's own biographies, *One Life* and *The Second Life*, were also very useful as source material.

Interviews are always vitally important and each one helps colour in the greater picture, especially when it is someone with direct knowledge of the affair. I am most grateful for the help and support of the following people (in no particular order): Deirdre Visser-Barnard, Kobus Visser, Tiaan Visser, Inéz Barnard, Adam Barnard, Andre Wagner, Karin Berman, Dene Friedmann, Tollie Lambrechts, Don Mackenzie, Joe de Nobrega, Rosemary Hickman, Anwar Mall, Otto Thaning, Susan Vosloo, David Cooper, Amanda Gouws, Peter Zilla, Johan Brink, Pieter Mulder, Pik and Ina Botha, Brian Astbury, Sigurd Olivier, Pamela Diamond, John Scott, Peter Hawthorne, Peet Simonis, Harry Shaw, Susan (Rossouw)

Tawse, Georgie (Hall) de Klerk, Alex and Jeremy Boraine and Karen Storay.

I would like to especially thank Piet Lötter and the Heart of Cape Town Museum for their support and kindness. Also the universities of Cape Town (in particular, Clive Kirkwood) and Stellenbosch, the Cape Town Medical Museum, as well as the universities of Stanford and Michigan, who assisted greatly in this book. Thanks, too, to those members of the Barnard family I have not mentioned by name, as well as the staff of the Beaufort West Museum led by Samantha Abselon, and archivists at Media24, in particular Colin Piers from *Huisgenoot* and Leonie Klootwyk from *Beeld* Biblioteek. I am also grateful to Waldimar Pelser, Yvonne Beyers and Willem Jordaan, the editors of *Rapport*, *Huisgenoot* and *Die Burger*, respectively, for their assistance. Old colleagues Bun Booyens and Aldi Schoeman are also owed a thank-you – their excellent book on *Die Burger*'s history was also used as a reference. The South African National Library and its staff were a great help, especially in finding rare books and old archive footage. I also made extensive use of the archives of the *Chicago Tribune, Der Spiegel*, the *Guardian* and the *Observer*.

I'd like to thank my research assistant, Amanda Hughes, and Jonathan Ball Publishers, in particular Ester Levinrad, who believed in the story from the start, and the editors behind the scenes who have done a great job. Friends like Jan-Jan, Paul and Sally, as well as Janet Heard and Jana Breytenbach, dankie. Also Siya, Debbie, Ewald, Jess, Dave, Monique, Peta, Chanel and the Birkenheart team, thanks.

Last, but not least by any means, to my family: thanks for the support and love, especially to dad Jimmy for the translating, ma Elna for the proofreading and pa Steyn for the support and advice. Jarrod, Justin and Germari you know what you mean to me. Sorry all for the late nights, cancelled weekends and holidays. My beautiful wife Marianne, without you it would be impossible and life would be just an endless cycle of meaningless routine. To the tractor- and reading-obsessed Alexander, one day I hope you'll enjoy this story too. We can't wait for your brother. Then the fun's going to really start. I love you all.

Author's note

I never met Christiaan Barnard and I was not there when the things that I describe in this book happened. I also never had the privilege to know many of the people about whom I write or quote from other sources. Every effort was made to contact each person who is still alive and plays a part in this book. Everyone, with few exceptions, was most accommodating and friendly. For that I am extremely grateful. The story is built on these interviews, as well as material I got from archives, libraries, books and museums, both in South Africa and the United States. I relied heavily on old correspondence and archival material, including from *The New York Times, Die Burger* and the *Cape Times*. The contributions from top heart surgeons, who gave of their valuable time to help with the more technical parts of this book, were also of great value. I hope they will forgive me for any technical errors. A lot of information was gathered, as well as many stories, more than could be included in this book. I am, however, happy with the end result and hope that everyone who helped me, especially the Barnard family, is too.

Sources

Barnard, Christiaan. (1977). *South Africa: Sharp Dissection*. Cape Town: Tafelberg.

Barnard, Christiaan. (1980). *Good Life, Good Death: A Doctor's Case for Euthanasia and Suicide*. Cape Town: Howard Timmins.

Barnard, Christiaan and Brewer, Chris (ed.). (1993). *Die Tweede Lewe*. Cape Town: Vlaeberg.

Barnard, Christiaan and Evans, Peter. (1984). *The Arthritis Handbook*. London: Michael Joseph.

Barnard, Christiaan and Molloy, Bob (ed.). (1984). *The Best of Barnard*. Cape Town: Molloy Publishers.

Barnard, Christiaan and Molloy, Bob (ed.). (1979). *The Best Medicine*. Cape Town: Tafelberg.

Barnard, Christiaan and Pepper, Curtis Bill. (1969). *Christiaan Barnard: One Life*. Cape Town: Tafelberg.

Barnard, Christiaan and Pepper, Curtis Bill. (1969). *Christiaan Barnard: Een Lewe*. Cape Town: Tafelberg.

Barnard, Deirdre. (2003). *Fat, Fame and Life with Father*. Cape Town: Double Storey.

Barnard, Deirdre. (2003). *Vet, Bekend en die Lewe Saam met Pa*. Cape Town: Double Storey.

Barnard, Louwtjie. (1971). *'n Hart Verwerp*. Cape Town: John Malherbe Edms Bpk.

Barnard, Marius and Johnson, Anthony. (1975). *Karoo*. Cape Town: Don Nelson.

Barnard, Marius with Norval, Simon. (2011). *Defining Moments: An Autobiography of Marius Barnard*. Cape Town: Zebra Press.

Blaiberg, Philip. (1969) *Looking at My Heart*. London: Heinemann.

Breytenbach, Breyten. (1984). *The True Confessions of an Albino Terrorist*. Paris: Farrar, Straus & Giroux.

Clingman, Stephen. (1998). *Bram Fischer: Afrikaner Revolutionary*. Amherst, MA: University of Massachusetts Press.

Coetzee, Pierre and Botha, Amanda. 'The Strange Hand of Fate in SA's Great Heart Drama'. *Scope* magazine, 29 December 1967.

Cooper, David (ed.) (1992). *Chris Barnard: By Those Who Know Him*. Cape Town: Vlaeberg.

Cooper, David. (2010). *Open Heart: The Radical Surgeons who Revolutionised Medicine.* New York: Kaplan Publishing.

Forrester, James. (2015). *The Heart Healers: The Misfits, Mavericks and Rebels who Created the Greatest Medical Breakthrough of Our Lives.* New York: St Martin's Press.

Hamilton, David. (2012). *A History of Organ Transplantation: Ancient Legends to Modern Practice.* Pittsburgh, PA: University of Pittsburgh Press.

Hawthorne, Peter. (1968). *The Transplanted Heart.* Johannesburg: Hugh Keartland Publishers.

Logan, Chris. (2003) *Celebrity Surgeon: Christiaan Barnard – A Life.* Cape Town: Jonathan Ball Publishers.

Malan, Marais. (1968). *Heart Transplant: The Story of Barnard and the Ultimate in Cardiac Surgery.* Johannesburg: Voortrekkerpers.

McRae, Donald. (2006). *Every Second Counts: The Race to Transplant the First Human Heart.* London: GP Putnam's Sons.

Pogrund, Benjamin. (2006). *How Can Man Die Better?* Cape Town: Jonathan Ball Publishers.

Naudé, Johan. (2007). *Making the Cut in South Africa: A Medico Political Story.* London: The Royal Society of Medicine Press.

Rhoodie, Eschel. (1983) *The Real Information Scandal.* London: Orbis.

Starzl, Thomas. (1992). *The Puzzle People: Memoirs of a Transplant Surgeon.* Pittsburgh, PA: University of Pittsburgh Press. (Accessed via University of Pittsburgh Press, Digital Editions).

Addditional sources

Archive footage. 'Netcare Christian Barnard Memorial Hospital: Opening Event', 2016. Accessed on YouTube. URL: https://goo.gl/oMeEF3.

Archive footage, 'Sandra op 'n Drafstap: Chris Barnard se Laaste Onderhoud', 2001. Accessed on YouTube. URL: https://goo.gl/R86CMe.

Altman, Lawrence K. (2001). 'Christiaan Barnard, 78, Surgeon For First Heart Transplant, Dies', *The New York Times.* URL: https://goo.gl/W2YwMf.

Ankney, Raymond N. (n.d.) 'Miracle in South Africa: A Historical Review of U.S. Magazines' Coverage of the First Heart Transplant'. University of North Carolina at Chapel Hill. URL: http://bit.ly/2rXpkKe.

Associated Press. (2003). 'James D Hardy, 84, Dies; Paved Way for Transplants', *The New York Times.* URL: https://goo.gl/hTzg5H.

Author unknown. (2001). 'End of era for *Cape Times* editor John Scott', *Cape Times.* URL: https://goo.gl/sTZ3yW.

Author unknown. (n.d.). 'A Heart Surgery Overview'. Texas Heart Institute. URL: http://www.texasheart.org/HIC/Topics/Proced/.

Author unknown. (n.d.). 'Cardiothoracic Surgery in South Africa'. Society of

Cardiothoracic Surgeons of South Africa. URL: http://www.sctssa.org/about-us/cardiothoracic-surgery-in-south-africa/

Author unknown. (2003). 'Obituary: James Hardy', *The Telegraph*. URL: https://goo.gl/c9jUbW.

Author unknown. (2007). 'Obituary: Sir Raymond Hoffenberg', *The Telegraph*. URL: http://bit.ly/2r3Tn30.

Author unknown. (n.d.). 'The Adrian Kantrowitz Papers'. US National Library of Medicine. URL: https://goo.gl/XQ8SMd.

Barker, Clyde and Markmann, James. (2013). 'Historical Overview of Transplantation', *Cold Spring Harbor Perspectives in Medicine*, 3(4). URL: https://goo.gl/1hJzBF.

Coulson, Alan S and Hanlon, Michael E (eds). (1997). 'War and the First Century of Heart Surgery', *Relevance: The Quarterly Journal of the Great War Society*, 6(1). URL: http://www.worldwar1.com/tgws/rel009.htm.

Goldstein, Susan. (1986). 'Miracle Man', *Orange Coast Magazine*. URL: http://bit.ly/2ruhdUf.

Hoffenberg, Raymond. (2001). 'Christiaan Barnard: His First Transplants and Their Impact on Concepts of Death', BMJ, 323(7327), 22 December, pp 1478–1480. URL: https://goo.gl/HGKhw5.

Hoffman, Jascha. (2008). 'Dr Adrian Kantrowitz, Cardiac Pioneer, Dies at 90', *The New York Times*. URL: https://goo.gl/oLW91Q.

London, David. (2007). 'Sir Raymond Hoffenberg: Exiled South African Physician and Campaigner for Medical Ethics'. Obituary, *The Guardian*. URL: http://bit.ly/2qjikdo.

Mitchell, James E, Crosby, Ross D, Wonderlich, Stephen A, and Adson, David E. (eds). (2000). *Elements of Clinical Research in Psychiatry*. Arlington, TX: American Psychiatric Association Publishing.

Morris, Peter J. (2012). 'Myburgh, Johannes Albertus (1928–2010)', Plarr's Lives of the Fellows Online. Royal College of Surgeons. URL: https://goo.gl/r3bMJ6.

Nathoo, Ayesha. (2009). *Hearts Exposed: Transplants and the Media in 1960s Britain*. London: Palgrave Macmillan.

Paget, Stephen. (1896). *The Surgery of the Chest*. Bristol: John Wright & Company.

Pearce, Jeremy. (2008). 'Richard Lower Dies at 78; Transplanted Animal and Human Hearts', *The New York Times*. URL: https://goo.gl/9MV9qw.

Simonis, Peet. (2012). 'Chris se Oorplanting: Die Storie Agter die Storie', *K'rant*. URL: http://bit.ly/2qjdTQ4.

Watts, Geoff. (2007). 'Obituary: Sir Raymond Hoffenberg', *The Lancet*, 369. URL: http://bit.ly/2r4XKN3.

Notes

Prologue
1. Author interview with Tollie Lambrechts.
2. Author interview with Susan (Rossouw) Tawse.

Chapter 1
1. Barnard, Marius and Johnson, Anthony. (1975). *Karoo*. Cape Town: Don Nelson.
2. Barnard, Louwtjie. (1971). *'n Hart Verwerp*. Cape Town: John Malherbe Edms Bpk.
3. Barnard, Marius with Norval, Simon. (2011). *Defining Moments: An Autobiography of Marius Barnard*. Cape Town: Zebra Press.
4. Ibid.
5. Ibid.
6. Ibid.
7. Barnard, Louwtjie. (1971). *'n Hart Verwerp*.
8. Johannes Barnard as recounted to *Die Burger* in 1967, *Die Burger* Archives.
9. Logan, Chris. (2003). *Celebrity Surgeon: Christiaan Barnard – A Life*. Cape Town: Jonathan Ball Publishers.
10. Barnard, Louwtjie. (1971). *'n Hart Verwerp*.
11. Johannes Barnard as recounted to *Die Burger* in 1967, *Die Burger* Archives.
12. Barnard, Louwtjie. (1971). *'n Hart Verwerp*.
13. Barnard, Christiaan and Molloy, Bob (ed.). (1984). *The Best of Barnard*. Cape Town: Molloy Publishers.
14. Ibid.
15. Barnard, Christiaan. (1977). *South Africa: Sharp Dissection*. Cape Town: Tafelberg.
16. Ibid.
17. Johannes Barnard as recounted to *Die Burger* in 1967, *Die Burger* Archives.

18. Barnard, Christiaan. (1977). *South Africa: Sharp Dissection*. Cape Town: Tafelberg.
19. Barnard, Louwtjie. (1971). *'n Hart Verwerp*.
20. Coetzee, Pierre and Botha, Amanda. 'The strange hand of fate in SA's great heart drama', *Scope* magazine, 29 December 1967.
21. Barnard, Louwtjie. (1971). *'n Hart Verwerp*.
22. Barnard, Christiaan. (1984). *The Best of Barnard*.
23. Ibid.
24. Barnard, Marius. (2011). *Defining Moments*.
25. Barnard, Louwtjie. (1971). *'n Hart Verwerp*.
26. Barnard, Marius. (2011). *Defining Moments*.
27. Johannes Barnard as recounted to *Die Burger* in 1967, *Die Burger* Archives.
28. Barnard, Marius. (2011). *Defining Moments*.
29. Ibid.
30. Barnard, Christiaan. (1980). *Good Life, Good Death: A Doctor's Case for Euthanasia and Suicide*. Cape Town: Howard Timmins.

Chapter 2

1. Barnard, Christiaan and Pepper, Curtis Bill. (1969). *Christiaan Barnard: One Life*. Cape Town: Tafelberg.
2. Blatchford, James W. (1985). 'Ludwig Rehn: The first successful cardiorrhaphy', *Annals of Thoracic Surgery*, 39(45), May, pp 492–495. http://www.annalsthoracicsurgery.org/article/S0003-4975(10)61972-8/pdf. See also Forrester, James. (2015). *The Heart Healers: The Misfits, Mavericks and Rebels who Created the Greatest Medical Breakthrough of Our Lives*. New York, St Martin's Press.
3. Ibid.
4. Barnard, Christiaan. (1969). *Christiaan Barnard: One Life*.
5. Barnard, Marius with Norval, Simon. (2011). *Defining Moments: An Autobiography of Marius Barnard*. Cape Town: Zebra Press.
6. Barnard, Christiaan. (1969). *Christiaan Barnard: One Life*.
7. Ibid.
8. Ibid.
9. Ibid.
10. Barnard, Christiaan with Evans, Peter. (1984). *The Arthritis Handbook*. London: Michael Joseph.
11. Barnard, Christiaan. (1969). *Christiaan Barnard: One Life*.
12. Ibid.
13. Barnard, Louwtjie. (1971). *'n Hart Verwerp*.
14. Ibid.
15. Ibid.
16. Barnard, Christiaan. (1969). *Christiaan Barnard: One Life*.

17. http://www.sctssa.org/about-us/cardi
18. Barnard, Christiaan. (1969). *Chris*
19. Ibid.
20. Barnard, Louwtjie. (1971). *'n Hart Verw*
21. Ibid.
22. Ibid.
23. Barnard, Christiaan. (1969). *Christiaan Barnar*
24. Ibid.
25. Barnard, Louwtjie. (1971). *'n Hart Verwerp.*
26. Barnard, Christiaan. (1969). *Christiaan Barnard: One L*
27. Cooper, David (ed.). (1992). *Chris Barnard: By Those Wh* Town: Vlaeberg.
28. Barnard, Louwtjie. (1971). *'n Hart Verwerp.*
29. Barnard, Christiaan. (1969). *Christiaan Barnard: One Life.*
30. Ibid.
31. Logan, Chris. (2003). *Celebrity Surgeon: Christiaan Barnard – A Life.* Jonathan Ball Publishers.
32. 'Chris Barnard: Heart of a Pioneer'. http://www.health24.com/Medical/Hea Heart-transplants/Chris-Barnard-profile-of-a-pioneer-20120721
33. Barnard, Christiaan. (1969). *Christiaan Barnard: One Life.*
34. Cooper, David (ed.) (1992). *Chris Barnard: By Those Who Know Him.*
35. Logan, Chris. (2003) *Celebrity Surgeon: Christiaan Barnard – A Life.*
36. Barnard, Louwtjie. (1971). *'n Hart Verwerp.*
37. Ibid.
38. Barnard, Marius. (2011). *Defining Moments.*
39. Barnard, Louwtjie. (1971). *'n Hart Verwerp.*
40. Barnard, Marius. (2011). *Defining Moments.*
41. Ibid.
42. Barnard, Christiaan. (1969). *Christiaan Barnard: One Life.*
43. Barnard, Deirdre. (2003). *Fat, Famous and Life with Father.* Cape Town: Double Storey.
44. Hawthorne, Peter. (1968). *The Transplanted Heart.* Johannesburg: Hugh Keartland Publishers.

Chapter 3

1. Coulson, Alan S and Hanlon, Michael E. (1997). 'War and the first century of heart surgery'. *Relevance: The Quarterly Journal of the Great War Society*, 6(1), Winter.
2. Ibid.
3. Ibid.
4. 'Dwight Emary Harken, MD, father and co-founder of Mended Hearts,

beat magazine, Spring 2014. http://www.mendedhearts.org/Docs/
.014.pdf.

Bruce. (1993). 'Dwight Harken, 83, the pioneer of surgery on the heart, is
ew York Times, 29 August.

, Alan S and Hanlon, Michael E. (1997). 'War and the first century of heart
y'.

ster, James. (2015). *The Heart Healers: The Misfits, Mavericks and Rebels
Created the Greatest Medical Breakthrough of our Lives*. New York, St
rtin's Press.

iner, Gerald. 'Pioneers in cardiac surgery: Dwight Emary Harken', taped
nterview. http://www.pbs.org/wgbh/nova/body/pioneers-heart-surgery.html.
Ibid.

Forrester, James. (2015). *The Heart Healers*.

. Nicol, A J, Navsaria, P H and Kahn, D. 'History of cardiac trauma
surgery'. *Continuing Medical Education*, 31(6), pp206-209, June 2013. http://www.
cmej.org.za/index.php/cmej/article/view/2756/2995.

12. 'Pioneers of heart surgery'. PBS.org NOVA, 4 April 1997. http://www.pbs.org/
wgbh/nova/body/pioneers-heart-surgery.html.

13. Coulson, Alan S and Hanlon, Michael. (1997).'War and the first century of heart
surgery'.

14. Rainer, Gerald. 'Pioneers in cardiac surgery: Dwight Emary Harken', taped
interview. http://www.pbs.org/wgbh/nova/body/pioneers-heart-surgery.html.

15. Ibid.

16. Ibid.

17. Ibid. Also, 'Surgeon C. Walton Lillehei Dies at 80'. *The Washington Post*, 8 July
1999. https://www.washingtonpost.com/.

18. 1987, Minneapolis, Associated Press, *Chicago Tribune* Archives.

19. Ibid.

20. 1987, Minneapolis, Associated Press, *Chicago Tribune* Archives.

21. Cooper, David. (2010). *Open Heart: The Radical Surgeons who Revolutionised
Medicine*. New York: Kaplan Publishing.

22. Ibid.

23. 'First Successful Open-Heart Surgery Patient Reunited with Doctor', Associated
Press, 13 August 1987.

24. Cohn, LH. (2003). 'Fifty years of open-heart surgery', *Circulation*, 107(17), pp
2168–70. http://circ.ahajournals.org/content/107/17/2168.

25. Ibid.

26. McRae, Donald. (2006). *Every Second Counts: The Race to Transplant the First
Human Heart*. London: GP Putnam's Sons.

27. Hawthorne, Peter. (1968). *The Transplanted Heart*. Johannesburg: Hugh Keartland
Publishers.

28. UCT Collections. http://atom.lib.uct.ac.za/index.php/chris-barnard-collection.

29. Barnard, Christiaan and Brewer, Chris (ed.). (1993). *Die Tweede Lewe*. Cape Town: Vlaeberg.
30. Ibid.
31. Altman, LK. (2001). 'Christiaan Barnard, 78, surgeon for first heart transplant, dies', *The New York Times*, 3 September. http://www.nytimes.com/2001/09/03/world/christiaan-barnard-78-surgeon-for-first-heart-transplant-dies.html.
32. Barnard, Christiaan and Pepper, Curtis Bill. (1969). *Christiaan Barnard: One Life*. Cape Town: Tafelberg.
33. Barnard, Christiaan and Molloy, Bob (ed.). (1984). *The Best of Barnard*. Cape Town: Molloy Publishers.
34. Barnard, Deirdre. (2003). *Fat, Fame and Life with Father*. Cape Town: Double Storey.
35. Ibid.
36. Ibid.
37. Barnard, Louwtjie. (1971). *'n Hart Verwerp*
38. McRae, Donald. (2006). *Every Second Counts*.
39. Barnard, Louwtjie. (1971) *'n Hart Verwerp*.
40. Cooper, David (ed.) (1992). *Chris Barnard: By Those Who Know Him*. Cape Town: Vlaeberg.
41. Barnard, Deirdre. (2003). *Fat, Fame and Life with Father*.
42. Barnard, Christiaan with Evans, Peter. (1984). *The Arthritis Handbook*. London: Michael Joseph.
43. Bridgstock, Graham. 'Interview with Chris Barnard'. *The Daily Mail*, 28 July 1998. http://www.apstherapy.com/about-aps-therapy/interview-with-chris-barnard.
44. Barnard, Christiaan. (1984). *The Arthritis Handbook*.
45. Ibid.
46. Ibid.
47. Barnard, Deirdre. (2003). *Fat, Fame and Life with Father*.
48. Ibid.
49. UCT Collections. http://atom.lib.uct.ac.za/index.php/chris-barnard-collection.
50. Cooper, David. (2010). *Open Heart: The Radical Surgeons who Revolutionised Medicine*.
51. Barnard, Christiaan and Molloy, Bob (ed.). (1984). *The Best of Barnard*. Cape Town: Molloy Publishers.
52. McRae, Donald. (2006). *Every Second Counts*.
53. Private correspondence of Dr Wangensteen in Heart of Cape Town Museum.
54. Barnard, Christiaan. (1969). *Christiaan Barnard: One Life*.

Chapter 4

1. Hawthorne, Peter. (1968). *The Transplanted Heart*. Johannesburg: Hugh Keartland Publishers.
2. UCT Archives.

3. Heart of Cape Town Museum.
4. Ibid.
5. Barnard, Christiaan and Pepper, Curtis Bill. (1969). *Christiaan Barnard: One Life.* Cape Town: Tafelberg.
6. Barnard, Christiaan, and Molloy, Bob (ed.). (1984). *The Best of Barnard.* Cape Town: Molloy Publishers.
7. CapeTalk podcast, Prof Anwar Mall, 13 January 2017. https://goo.gl/3k6VnA. Also, author interview with Prof Anwar Mall in Cape Town, February-March 2017.
8. Heart of Cape Town Museum.
9. Ibid.
10. Barnard, Christiaan and Molloy, Bob (ed.). (1984). *The Best of Barnard.*
11. Barnard, Christiaan. (1969). *Christiaan Barnard: One Life.*
12. Barnard, Christiaan and Molloy, Bob (ed.). (1984). *The Best of Barnard.*
13. Barnard, Louwtjie. (1971). *'n Hart Verwerp.* Cape Town: John Malherbe.
14. Ibid.
15. Barnard, Johannes. Articles he wrote for *Die Burger*, December 1967.
16. Ibid.
17. Ibid.
18. Barnard, Louwtjie. (1971). *'n Hart Verwerp.*
19. Barnard, Christiaan. (1969). *Christiaan Barnard: One Life.*
20. Barnard, Louwtjie. (1971). *'n Hart Verwerp.*
21. Ibid.
22. Hawthorne, Peter. (1968). *The Transplanted Heart.*
23. Barnard, Christiaan. (1969). *Christiaan Barnard: One Life.*
24. Ibid.
25. Ibid.
26. Ibid.
27. Ibid.
28. Ibid.
29. Netcare Christiaan Barnard Exhibition, Heart of Cape Town Museum.
30. SA National Library Archives, *Cape Times*, 30 July 1958.
31. Netcare Christiaan Barnard Exhibition, Heart of Cape Town Museum.
32. Barnard, Christiaan. (1984). *The Best of Barnard.*
33. Ibid.
34. Cotton, Michael, Hickman, Rosemary and Suleman Mall, Anwar. (2014). 'Hamilton Naki, his life and his role in the first heart transplant.' *The Royal College of Surgeons of England Bulletin*, 96: 224–227. https://goo.gl/rXCyvG. Also, Barnard, Deirdre. (2003). Fat, Fame and Life with Father.
35. Author interview with Prof Rosemary Hickman. Also, Barnard, Marius with Norval, Simon. (2011). *Defining Moments.*
36. Author interview with Hendrik Snyders, the Springbok Experience Rugby Museum, Cape Town, 31 May 2017. Also, Barnard, Marius with Norval, Simon.

(2011) *Defining Moments*. Cape Town: Zebra Press.

37. Barnard, Deirdre. (2003). *Fat, Fame and Life with Father*.
38. 'Hamilton Naki, an unrecognised surgical pioneer, died on May 29th, aged 78', *Economist* Obituary, 9 June 2005. http://www.economist.com/node/4054912
39. CapeTalk podcast, Prof Anwar Mall, 13 January 2017. https://goo.gl/3k6VnA. Also, author interview with Prof Anwar Mall in Cape Town, February-March 2017.
40. *Economist* Correction, 9 June 2005. http://www.economist.com/node/4174683.
41. Ibid.
42. Terblanche, John. 'Letter to the Editor'. *South African Medical Journal*, 95 (8), August 2005. http://www.samj.org.za/index.php/samj/article/viewFile/1765/1090.
43. Ibid.
44. Ibid.
45. Interview with Prof Rosemary Hickman. Also CapeTalk podcast, Prof Anwar Mall, 13 January 2017. www.702.co.za.
46. Ibid.
47. Hawthorne, Peter. (1968). *The Transplanted Heart*.
48. Barnard, Deirdre. (2003). *Fat, Fame and Life with Father*.

Chapter 5

1. 'James D Hardy, 84, dies; paved way for transplants', Associated Press, 21 February 2003. https://goo.gl/hTzg5H.
2. Cooper, David. (2010). *Open Heart: The Radical Surgeons who Revolutionised Medicine*. New York: Kaplan Publishing.
3. Lehew, Dudley. (1964). 'Substitute heart works for an hour in historic surgery', *Utica Daily Press*, Associated Press, 25 January. https://goo.gl/GHEsLp.
4. Cooper, David. (2010). *Open Heart: The Radical Surgeons who Revolutionised Medicine*.
5. Ibid.
6. Ibid.
7. *Time* magazine, 7 January 1955. https://goo.gl/5wwMoe.
8. Pace, Eric. 'Vladimir P Demikhov, 82, pioneer in transplants, dies', 25 November 1998. https://goo.gl/eixroR.
9. Ibid.
10. 'At the cutting edge of the impossible: A tribute to Vladimir P Demikhov, a pioneer of organ transplantation'. *Transplant Proc*, 43(4), pp1221–1, May 2011.
11. Ibid.
12. *The New York Times* Archives.
13. Ibid.
14. 'At the cutting edge of the impossible: A tribute to Vladimir P Demikhov, a pioneer of organ transplantation'. *Transplant Proc*, 43(4), pp1221–1, May 2011.
15. Malan, Marais. (1968). *Heart Transplant: The Story of Barnard and the Ultimate*

in Cardiac Surgery. Johannesburg: Voortrekkerpers.

16. 'At the cutting edge of the impossible: A tribute to Vladimir P. Demikhov, a pioneer of organ transplantation.'. *Transplant Proc*, 43(4), pp1221–1, May 2011

17. Malan, Marais. (1968). *Heart Transplant: The Story of Barnard and the Ultimate in Cardiac Surgery.*

18. McRae, Donald. (2006). *Every Second Counts.* London: GP Putnam's Sons.

19. Langer, Rob.'Vladimir P. Demikhov, a pioneer of organ transplantation.' *Transplant Proe*, 43(4), pp 1221–2, May 2011 https://www.ncbi.nlm.nih.gov/pubmed/21620094.

20. *The New York Times* Archives.

21. Ibid.

22. Ibid. Also, Pearce, Jeremy. 'Richard Lower dies at 78; transplanted animal and human hearts.' 31 May 2008. https://goo.gl/9MV9qw.

23. *The New York Times* Archives.

24. Pearce, Jeremy. 'Richard Lower dies at 78; transplanted animal and human hearts.'

25. Adrian Kantrowitz. US National Library of Medicine: The Adrian Kantrowitz Papers. https://goo.gl/XQ8SMd.

26. *The New York Times* Archives.

27. Adrian Kantrowitz. US National Library of Medicine: The Adrian Kantrowitz Papers.

28. Hoffenberg, Raymond. (2001). 'Christiaan Barnard: His first transplants and their impact on concepts of death', *BMJ*, 323(7327), 22 December, pp 1478–1480. https://goo.gl/YkmNm8.

29. Ibid.

30. Malan, Marais. (1968). *Heart Transplant: The Story of Barnard and the Ultimate in Cardiac Surgery.*

Chapter 6

1. Barker, Clyde, and Markmann, James. (2013). 'Historical overview of transplantation', *Cold Spring Harbor Perpectives in Medicine*, 3(4). https://goo.gl/1hJzBF.

2. Heart of Cape Town Museum.

3. Netcare, Christiaan Barnard Memorial Hospital Exhibition, Joe de Nobrega Collection. Author interview with Joe de Nobrega, Cape Town, August 2017.

4. Netcare, Christiaan Barnard Memorial Hospital Exhibition. Also, History of the Chris Barnard Division of Cardiothoracic Surgery. https://goo.gl/pTvG61.

5. Goosen, Carl. (2014). 'One critical medical device: Aortic valve prosthesis — The inventor perspective on design.' https://goo.gl/n5ZjDF

6. Ibid.

7. Bolognesi, Natasha. (2007) 'The transplant timeline', Heart of Cape Town Museum.

8. Netcare, Christiaan Barnard Memorial Hospital Exhibition. Also, History of the Chris Barnard Division of Cardiothoracic Surgery.

9. Barnard, Marius, with Norval, Simon. (2011) *Defining Moments*. Cape Town: Zebra Press.

10. Cooper, David. (2010). *Open Heart: The Radical Surgeons who Revolutionised Medicine*. New York: Kaplan Publishing.

11. Hawthorne, Peter. (1968). *The Transplanted Heart*. Johannesburg: Hugh Keartland Publishers.

12. Heart of Cape Town Museum.

13. Cooper, David. (2010). *Open Heart: The Radical Surgeons who Revolutionised Medicine*.

14. Ibid.

15. *The New York Times* Archives.

16. Hawthorne, Peter. (1968). *The Transplanted Heart*. Johannesburg: Hugh Keartland Publishers.

17. Personal correspondence with Owen Wangensteen at Heart of Cape Town Museum.

18. Horwitz, Simonne. 'Half a century: A brief history of kidney transplantation in Johannesburg'. 17 January 2017. *Mail&Guardian*. http://mg.co.za/article/2017-01-17-half-a-century-a-brief-history-of-kidney-transplantation-in-johannesburg.

19. Myburgh, JA. (1980). 'Transplantation: The Johannesburg experience', *South African Medical Journal*, 19 April.

20. Starzl, Thomas. (1992). *The Puzzle People: Memoirs of a Transplant Surgeon*. Pittsburgh, PA: University of Pittsburgh Press.

21. Ibid.

22. Horwitz, Simonne. 'Half a century: A brief history of kidney transplantation in Johannesburg.'

23. Morris, Peter J. 'Myburgh, Johannes Albertus (1928-2010)'. (2012). https://livesonline.rcseng.ac.uk/biogs/E002852b.htm.

24. Cooper, David. (2010). *Open Heart: The Radical Surgeons who Revolutionised Medicine*.

25. Barnard, Marius. (2011). *Defining Moments*.

26. Barnard, Christiaan and Pepper, Curtis Bill. (1969). *Christiaan Barnard: One Life*. Cape Town: Tafelberg.

27. McRae, Donald. (2006). *Every Second Counts*. London: GP Putnam's Sons.

28. Barnard, Christiaan. (1969). *Christiaan Barnard: One Life*.

29. Starzl, Thomas. (1992). *The Puzzle People: Memoirs of a Transplant Surgeon*.

30. Heart of Cape Town Museum.

31. McRae, Donald. (2006). *Every Second Counts*.

32. Ibid.

33. Cooper, David. (2010). *Open Heart: The Radical Surgeons who Revolutionised Medicine*.

34. Heart of Cape Town Museum.
35. *Huisgenoot*, 19 January 1968.
36. Ibid.
37. Archive material: *Die Burger, Huisgenoot, Scope.*
38. *Huisgenoot*, 19 January 1968.
39. Heart of Cape Town Museum.
40. Ibid.
41. Barnard, Christiaan. (1969). *Christiaan Barnard: One Life.*
42. Heart of Cape Town Museum.
43. 'The first heart transplant: The Jewish connection', *Southern Africa Jewish Genealogy, Special Interest Group* (SA-SIG), 2(6), March 2002.
44. Cooper, David (ed.). (1992). *Chris Barnard: By Those Who Know Him.* Cape Town: Vlaeberg.
45. Ibid.
46. Ibid. Also Heart of Cape Town Museum.
47. Barnard, Christiaan. (1969). *Christiaan Barnard: One Life.*
48. Hawthorne, Peter. (1968). *The Transplanted Heart.*
49. Barnard, Christiaan. (1969). *Christiaan Barnard: One Life*
50. Cooper, David (ed.). (1992). *Chris Barnard: By Those Who Know Him.*
51. Heart of Cape Town Museum. Also, Hawthorne, Peter. (1968). *The Transplanted Heart.*
52. Barnard, Marius. (2011). *Defining Moments.*
53. Ibid.
54. Malan, Marais. (1968). *Heart Transplant: The Story of Barnard and the Ultimate in Cardiac Surgery.* Johannesburg: Voortrekkerpers.
55. Ibid.
56. Ibid.
57. Barnard, Marius. (2011). *Defining Moments.*
58. McRae, Donald. (2006). *Every Second Counts.*
59. *Der Spiegel* Online Archives.
60. Malan, Marais. (1968). *Heart Transplant: The Story of Barnard and the Ultimate in Cardiac Surgery.*
61. *Der Spiegel* Online Archives.
62. Barnard, Christiaan. (1969). *Christiaan Barnard: One Life.*
63. Hawthorne, Peter. (1968). *The Transplanted Heart.*
64. Ibid.

Chapter 7

1. Green, David B. (2013). '1967: First heart transplant patient goes under the knife', *Jewish World*, 3 December. https://goo.gl/NVNDYn.
2. Barnard, Christiaan and Pepper, Curtis Bill. (1969). *Christiaan Barnard: One Life.* Cape Town: Tafelberg.

3. Ibid.
4. Ibid.
5. Ibid.
6. Heart of Cape Town Museum.
7. Green, David B. (2013). '1967: First heart transplant patient goes under the knife'.
8. *The New York Times* Archives, 25 December 1967.
9. Green, David B. (1967). 'First heart transplant patient goes under the knife'.
10. Brits, Elsabé. (2014). 'Vergete Hartseer van Eerste Hartoorplanting', *Die Burger*, 17 January.
11. Ibid.
12. Coetzee, Pierre and Botha, Amanda. (1967). 'The strange hand of fate in SA's great heart drama', *Scope* magazine, 29 December.
13. Brits, Elsabé. (2014). 'Vergete hartseer van eerste hartoorplanting', *Die Burger*, 17 January.
14. Coetzee, Pierre and Botha, Amanda. (1967). 'The strange hand of fate in SA's great heart drama', *Scope* magazine.

Chapter 8

1. Malan, Marais. (1968). *Heart Transplant: The Story of Barnard and the Ultimate in Cardiac Surgery*. Johannesburg: Voortrekkerpers.
2. Ibid.
3. Ibid.
4. Cooper, David (ed.). (1992). *Chris Barnard: By Those Who Know Him*. Cape Town: Vlaeberg.
5. Ibid.
6. Ibid.
7. Malan, Marais. (1968). *Heart Transplant: The Story of Barnard and the Ultimate in Cardiac Surgery*.
8. Cooper, David (ed.). (1992). *Chris Barnard: By Those Who Know Him*.
9. Ibid.
10. 'The Operation. A Human Cardiac Transplant: An interim report of a successful operation performed at Groote Schuur Hospital, Cape Town.' *South African Medical Journal*, 30 December 1967.
11. Cooper, David (ed.). (1992). *Chris Barnard: By Those Who Know Him*.
12. Barnard, Marius, and Norval, Simon. (2011). *Defining Moments*. Cape Town: Zebra Press.
13. *Cape Times*, 4 December 1967.
14. National Library: *Cape Times* Archives.
15. *Cape Times*, 4 December 1967.
16. Ibid.
17. Brits, Elsabé. (2014). 'Vergete hartseer van eerste hartoorplanting', *Die Burger*, 17 January 2014.

18. Ibid.
19. Johannes Barnard as recounted to *Die Burger* in 1967. *Die Burger* Archives.
20. Heart of Cape Town Museum.

Chapter 9

1. Archive footage per 2016 Netcare video. Accessed on YouTube. https://goo.gl/oMeEF3.
2. Ibid.
3. Barnard, Marius, and Norval, Simon. (2011). *Defining Moments*. Cape Town: Zebra Press.
4. Heart of Cape Town Museum.
5. University of Minnesota Archives. Wangensteen Correspondence.
6. Heart of Cape Town Museum.
7. Ibid.
8. From Sapa-Reuter article in the *Cape Times*, 6 December 1967.
9. Ibid.
10. *Die Huisgenoot*, 19 January 1968.
11. Cooper, David. (2010). *Open Heart: The Radical Surgeons who Revolutionised Medicine*. New York: Kaplan Publishing.
12. Malan, Marais. (1968). *Heart Transplant: The Story of Barnard and the Ultimate in Cardiac Surgery*. Johannesburg: Voortrekkerpers. Also, *The New York Times* Archives.
13. *The New York Times* Archives.
14. Ibid.
15. Ibid.
16. Ibid.
17. Donald McRae, Tuesday, 18 November 2008. http://bit.ly/2r33q8w.
18. Ibid.
19. Malan, Marais. (1968). *Heart Transplant: The Story of Barnard and the Ultimate in Cardiac Surgery*.
20. Hoffman, Jascha. (2008). 'Dr Adrian Kantrowitz, cardiac pioneer, dies at 90', 19 November 2008. https://goo.gl/oLW91Q.
21. Archive footage per 2016 Netcare video. Accessed on YouTube. https://goo.gl/oMeEF3.
22. *Time* magazine, 22 December 1967.
23. Ibid.
24. Ibid.
25. Ibid.
26. *Time* magazine, 29 December 1967.
27. Malan, Marais. (1968). *Heart Transplant: The Story of Barnard and the Ultimate in Cardiac Surgery*.

28. Ibid.
29. Ibid.
30. Goldstein, Susan. (1986). 'Miracle man', *Orange Coast Magazine*. http://bit.ly/2ruhdUf.
31. *Time* magazine, 29 December 1967.
32. Barnard, Marius. (2011). *Defining Moments*.
33. Brits, Elsabé. (2014). 'Vergete hartseer van eerste hartoorplanting', *Die Burger*, 17 January.

Chapter 10
1. Barnard, Louwtjie. (1971). *'n Hart Verwerp*. Cape Town: John Malherbe.
2. Cooper, David (ed.). (1992). *Chris Barnard: By Those Who Know Him*. Cape Town: Vlaeberg.
3. Ibid.
4. Ibid.
5. *The New York Times* Archives.
6. Barnard, Louwtjie. (1971). *'n Hart Verwerp*.
7. Ibid.
8. *The New York Times* Archives.
9. Malan, Marais. (1968). *Heart Transplant: The Story of Barnard and the Ultimate in Cardiac Surgery*. Johannesburg: Voortrekkerpers.
10. Blaiberg, Philip. (1969). *Looking at My Heart*. London: Heinemann.
11. Ibid.
12. Ibid.
13. Ibid.
14. Ibid.
15. Ibid.
16. Ibid.
17. Malan, Marais. (1968). *Heart Transplant: The Story of Barnard and the Ultimate in Cardiac Surgery*.
18. Blaiberg, Philip. (1969). *Looking at My Heart*.
19. Ibid.
20. Malan, Marais. (1968). *Heart Transplant: The Story of Barnard and the Ultimate in Cardiac Surgery*.
21. Malan, Marais. (1968). *Heart Transplant: The Story of Barnard and the Ultimate in Cardiac Surgery*. Also, *Cape Times*, 3 January 1968.
22. Hoffenberg, Raymond. (2001). 'Christiaan Barnard: His first transplants and their impact on concepts of death', *BMJ*, 323(7327), 22 December, pp 1478–1480. https://goo.gl/YkmNm8.
23. Barnard, Christiaan, and Brewer, Chris (ed.). (1993). *Die Tweede Lewe*. Cape Town: Vlaeberg.

24. Barnard, Christiaan, and Evans, Peter. (1984). *The Arthritis Handbook*. London: Michael Joseph.
25. *Cape Times*, 3 January 1968.
26. Blaiberg, Philip. (1969). *Looking at My Heart*. Also, Malan, Marais. (1968). *Heart Transplant: The Story of Barnard and the Ultimate in Cardiac Surgery*.
27. Olivier, Sigurd. The King of Hearts blog. http://www.magicmirror.nl/newfiles/shenanigans-1.html. Sigurd Olivier's two photographic books, *Gentlewoman* and *Touch Love*, the first an ode to femininity, the latter on lovemaking, were banned in South Africa, but had success internationally. He has recently completed a biographical novel in which the Blaiberg account plays a part.
28. Royal College of Physicians. Reuben Mibashan Biography. https://goo.gl/6aPjst.

Chapter 11

1. *The New York Times* Archives.
2. 'norman Shumway, heart transplantation pioneer, dies at 83'. Stanford Archives. https://goo.gl/P4Y3nZ.
3. *The New York Times* Archives.
4. 'norman Shumway, heart transplantation pioneer, dies at 83'. Stanford Archives.
5. Adrian Kantrowitz. US National Library of Medicine: The Adrian Kantrowitz Papers. https://goo.gl/XQ8SMd.
6. Hoffman, Jascha. (2008). 'Dr Adrian Kantrowitz, cardiac pioneer, dies at 90', 19 November. https://goo.gl/oLW91Q.
7. McRae, Donald. (2006). *Every Second Counts*. London: GP Putnam's Sons.
8. Naudé, Johan. (2007). *Making the Cut in South Africa: A Medico Political Story*. London: The Royal Society of Medicine Press.
9. Barnard, Christiaan, and Brewer, Chris (ed.). (1993). *Die Tweede Lewe*. Cape Town: Vlaeberg.
10. Ibid.
11. Ibid.
12. Barnard, Christiaan. (1993). *Die Tweede Lewe*.
13. *The New York Times* Archives.

Chapter 12

1. 'Lord God, it beats again', *Der Spiegel*, 4 March 1968.
2. Barnard, Louwtjie. (1971). *'n Hart Verwerp*. Cape Town: John Malherbe.
3. Goldstein, Susan. (1986). 'Miracle man', *Orange Coast Magazine*. http://bit.ly/2ruhdUf.
4. *The New York Times* Archives.
5. Barnard, Louwtjie. (1971). *'n Hart Verwerp*.
6. Cooper, David. (2010). *Open Heart: The Radical Surgeons who Revolutionised*

Medicine. New York: Kaplan Publishing.

7. *The Guardian/Observer* Digital Archives.

8. Mitchell, James E, Crosby, Ross D et al (ed's.). (2000). *Elements of Clinical Research in Psychiatry*. New York: American Psychiatric Association Publishing.

9. Jonsen, Albert R. (2003). *The Birth of Bioethics*. New York: Oxford University Press.

10. Ibid.

11. *The New York Times* Archives.

12. Barnard, Christiaan. (1977). *South Africa: Sharp Dissection*. Cape Town: Tafelberg.

13. Goldstein, Susan. (1986). 'Miracle man', *Orange Coast Magazine*.

14. Hamilton, David. (2012). *A History of Organ Transplantation: Ancient Legends to Modern Practice*. Pittsburgh, PA: University of Pittsburgh Press.

15. Jonsen, Albert R. (1998). *The Birth of Bioethics*.

16. Hamilton, David. (2012). *A History of Organ Transplantation*.

17. *The New York Times* Archives.

18. Ibid. Also, Ankey, Raymond N. 'Miracle in South Africa: A historical review of US magazines' coverage of the first heart transplant'. University of North Carolina at Chapel Hill. http://bit.ly/2rXpkKe.

19. Barnard, Christiaan, and Brewer, Chris (ed.). (1993). *Die Tweede Lewe*. Cape Town: Vlaeberg.

20. *The New York Times* Archives.

21. 'Heart transplants: The longest survivor'. Associated Press archive footage, accessed on YouTube. https://www.youtube.com/watch?v=n8ohEArw-N0.

22. Ibid.

23. Ibid.

24. *The New York Times* Archives.

25. Ibid.

26. *Chicago Tribune*, 12 October 1969.

27. *The New York Times* Archives.

Chapter 13

1. 'Dr Barnard marries Barbara Zoellner, 19', Special edition, *The New York Times*, 14 February 1970.

2. 'Dr Barnard weds socialite, 19, in early Valentine Day vows', *Chicago Tribune*, 14 February 1970.

3. Ibid.

4. Ibid.

5. Ibid.

6. 'Barnard and Bride', *Chicago Tribune*, 17 February 1970.

7. Hassoulas, Joannis. 'Transplantation of the heart: An overview of 40 years' clinical

and research experience at Groote Schuur Hospital and the University of Cape Town: Part II. Laboratory Research Experience', *South African Medical Journal*, 102 (6.2), March 2012. http://www.ncbi.n/m.ni.gov/pubmed/22668901.

8. *The New York Times* Archives.
9. *The Guardian/Observer* Digital Archives.
10. Hassoulas, Joannis. (2011). 'Transplantation of the heart'.
11. Media clippings in Archives, Associated Press.
12. Cooper, David. (2010). *Open Heart: The Radical Surgeons who Revolutionised Medicine*. New York: Kaplan Publishing.
13. The *Guardian/Observer* Digital Archives.
14. Cooper, David. (2010). *Open Heart: The Radical Surgeons who Revolutionised Medicine*.
15. Ibid.
16. Brink, Johan, and Hassoulas, Joannis. (2009). 'The first human heart transplant and further advances in cardiac transplantation at Groote Schuur Hospital and the University of Cape Town', *Cardiovascular Journal of Africa*, 20 (1), January/ February.
17. Cooper, David. (2010). *Open Heart: The Radical Surgeons who Revolutionised Medicine*.
18. UCT Archives.
19. Clippings in the UCT Christiaan Barnard Collection. 'Dr Barnard sees duty to do heart transplants'. *London Times*, 2 May 1972.
20. Cooper, David (ed.). (1992). *Chris Barnard: By Those Who Know Him*. Cape Town: Vlaeberg. Also, UCT Archives.
21. Cooper, David (ed.). (1992). *Chris Barnard: By Those Who Know Him*.
22. Ibid.
23. *The Guardian/Observer* Digital Archives.
24. Cooper, David (ed.). (1992). *Chris Barnard: By Those Who Know Him*.
25. United Press International News Clippings, 23 April 1975.
26. Hassoulas, Joannis. (2011). 'Transplantation of the heart'.
27. Ibid.
28. Wright, Robin. 'Barnard: Baboon Heart Couldn't Handle Demands.' *The Washington Post*, 22 June 1977.
29. Cooper, David (ed.). (1992). *Chris Barnard: By Those Who Know Him*.
30. Ibid.
31. Ibid.
32. Barnard, Christiaan, and Molloy, Bob (ed.). (1984). *The Best of Barnard*. Cape Town: Molloy Publishers.
33. Ibid.
34. Ibid.

Chapter 14

1. *The New York Times* Archives.
2. Ibid.
3. *The Guardian/Observer* Digital Archives.
4. Ibid.
5. Ibid.
6. *The New York Times* Archives.
7. *Die Burger*, 30 June 1973.
8. UCT Archives.
9. *The Guardian/Observer* Digital Archives.
10. Ibid.
11. Interviews with Don Mackenzie in 2017.
12. *The New York Times* Archives.
13. Ibid.
14. Barnard, Christiaan, and Brewer, Chris (ed.). (1993). *Die Tweede Lewe*. Cape Town: Vlaeberg.
15. Ibid.

Chapter 15

1. Barnard, Christiaan, and Brewer, Chris (ed.). (1993). *Die Tweede Lewe*. Cape Town: Vlaeberg.
2. Rhoodie, Eschel. (1983). *The Real Information Scandal*. London: Orbis.
3. Brink, Johan and Hassoulas, Joannis. (2009). 'The first human heart transplant and further advances in cardiac transplantation at Groote Schuur Hospital and the University of Cape Town', *Cardiovascular Journal of Africa*, 20 (1), January/February.
4. Pogrund, Benjamin. (2006). *How Can Man Die Better?* Cape Town: Jonathan Ball Publishers.
5. Ibid.
6. Ibid.
7. Ibid.
8. Barnard, Marius, with Norval, Simon. (2011) *Defining Moments*. Cape Town: Zebra Press.
9. Ibid.
10. Pogrund, Benjamin. (2006). *How Can Man Die Better?*
11. Ibid.
12. Barnard, Marius. (2011) *Defining Moments*.
13. Ibid.
14. Barnard, Christiaan. (1993). *Die Tweede Lewe*.
15. Barnard, Marius. (2011) *Defining Moments*.
16. De Nobrega recording, Netcare Exhibition, Netcare Christiaan Barnard Memorial

Hospital, Cape Town. Also, author interview with De Nobrega.

17. Pogrund, Benjamin. (2006). *How Can Man Die Better?*
18. Barnard, Christiaan. (1993). *Die Tweede Lewe.*
19. Barnard, Marius. (2011) *Defining Moments*
20. Suzman, Helen. (1993). *In No Uncertain Terms: A South African Memoir.* London: Alfred A Knopf.
21. Pogrund, Benjamin. (2006). *How Can Man Die Better?*
22. Ibid.
23. Barnard, Christiaan. (1993). *Die Tweede Lewe.*
24. *The Guardian/Observer* Digital Archive.
25. Ibid.
26. 'Prof. Barnard by Breyten in sel', *Huisgenoot*, 23 December 1977.
27. Ibid.
28. Barnard, Christiaan. (1993). *Die Tweede Lewe.*
29. Breytenbach, Breyten. (1984). *The True Confessions of an Albino Terrorist.* Paris: Farrar, Straus & Giroux.
30. Ibid.
31. Ibid.
32. Ibid.
33. Barnard, Christiaan, and Molloy, Bob (ed.). (1984). *The Best of Barnard.* Cape Town: Molloy Publishers.
34. Interview with Pieter Mulder, March 2017.
35. Barnard, Christiaan. (1993). *Die Tweede Lewe.*
36. Letter from Dr Francis Ames to Chris Barnard, August 1980. Beaufort West Museum Archives.
37. Correspondence, Beaufort West Museum Archives.

Chapter 16

1. Cooper, David (ed.). (1992). *Chris Barnard: By Those Who Know Him.* Cape Town: Vlaeberg.
2. Barnard, Christiaan, and Brewer, Chris (ed.). (1993). *Die Tweede Lewe.* Cape Town: Vlaeberg.
3. Ibid.
4. Ibid.
5. Ibid.
6. Ibid. Also multiple author interviews with Deirdre Barnard and Dene Friedmann.
7. Ibid.
8. Cooper, David (ed.). (1992). *Chris Barnard: By Those Who Know Him..* Also author interviews with Deirdre Barnard and Dene Friedmann.
9. Bridgstock, Graham. (1998). 'Interview with Chris Barnard'. *The Daily Mail.* http://www.apstherapy.com/about-aps-therapy/interview-with-chris-barnard.

10. Matchan, Linda. Interview with Christiaan Barnard. *Maclean's Magazine*, 9 January 1978.
11. Barnard, Christiaan. (1993). *Die Tweede Lewe.*
12. Hawthorne, Peter. 'His hands stiffened by arthritis, Christiaan Barnard explores a second career in television', 17 April 1978. https://goo.gl/UNUg61.
13. Bridgstock, Graham. (1998). 'Interview with Chris Barnard'. *The Daily Mail.* http://www.apstherapy.com/about-aps-therapy/interview-with-chris-barnard.
14. Barnard, Christiaan, and Evans, Peter. (1984). *The Arthritis Handbook*. London: Michael Joseph.
15. Ibid.
16. Barnard, Deirdre. (2003). *Fat, Fame and Life with Father*. Cape Town: Double Storey.
17. Barnard, Christiaan, and Molloy, Bob (ed.). (1984). *The Best of Barnard*. Cape Town: Molloy Publishers.
18. Ibid.
19. 'Christiaan Barnard's son found dead in bathtub', *Chicago Tribune*, 1 February 1984. https://goo.gl/KSFgdo.
20. Ibid.
21. 'Dr Christiaan Barnard's son found dead', 1 March 1984. https://goo.gl/yTwnzz.
22. 'Christiaan Barnard's son found dead in bathtub', *Chicago Tribune.*
23. Barnard, Christiaan. (1984). *The Best of Barnard.*
24. Ibid.
25. Ibid.
26. Ibid.
27. Logan, Chris. (2003) *Celebrity Surgeon: Christiaan Barnard – A Life*. Cape Town: Jonathan Ball Publishers.
28. Barnard, Deirdre. (2003). *Fat, Fame and Life with Father*. Also, 'Christiaan Barnard's son found dead in bathtub', *Chicago Tribune.*
29. 'Drug That Reduces Risk In Transplants Gets Early Approval'. *The New York Times*, 3 September 1983, http://www.nytimes.com. Also, Upton, Harriet. 'Origin of drugs in current use: the cyclosporine story'. (2001). http://www.davidmoore.org.uk/Sec04_01.htm
30. Pearce, Jeremy. 'Richard Lower dies at 78; transplanted animal and human hearts', 31 May 2008. https://goo.gl/9MV9qw.
31. Mieny, CJ. (1988). 'Die huidige status van orgaanoorplantings'. Department of Surgery, University of Pretoria and the H. Verwoerd Hospital.
32. 'Dr Barnard's new elixir of youth', *New York Magazine*, 18 November 1985.
33. Lauerman, Connie. 'Why Christiaan Barnard fronts for Glycel'. *Chicago Tribune*, 16 April 1986, www.chicagotribune.newspapers.com.
34. 'Dr Barnard's new elixir of youth', *New York Magazine.*
35. Lauerman, Connie. 'Why Christiaan Barnard fronts for Glycel'.
36. 'Dr Barnard's new elixir of youth', *New York Magazine.*

37. Lauerman, Connie. 'Why Christiaan Barnard fronts for Glycel', *Chicago Tribune*.
38. Ibid.
39. Greer, William. 'Doctor's Role in Cosmetics Ads Criticized', *The New York Times*, 7 March 1986. http://goo.gl/EvUVkU.
40. Barnard, Christiaan. (1993). *Die Tweede Lewe*.
41. Greer, William. 'Doctor's Role in Cosmetics Ads Criticized', *The New York Times*.
42. Ibid.
43. Ibid.
44. 'Dr Barnard's new elixir of youth', *New York Magazine*.

Chapter 17

1. 'Christiaan Barnard, Model Wed', Associated Press, 24 January 1988. https://goo.gl/A2TcgA.
2. Ibid.
3. Barnard, Christiaan, and Brewer, Chris (ed.). (1993). *Die Tweede Lewe*. Cape Town: Vlaeberg.
4. Cooper, David (ed.). (1992). *Chris Barnard: By Those Who Know Him*. Cape Town: Vlaeberg.
5. Ibid.
6. Dougherty, Steven. 'Lion in winter', *People*, 8 April 1996. https://goo.gl/vGRhcW.
7. Christiaan Barnard Heart Foundation.
8. Otto Thaning, multiple interviews with author in 2017.
9. Ellison, Sarah. (2013). 'Diana's impossible dream', *Vanity Fair*, September 2013. https://goo.gl/hDb9TD.
10. Ibid.
11. Feiden, Douglas. 'Dodi, not Di's love, doctor stole her heart, book says', *New York Daily News*, 12 August 1999. https://goo.gl/ykxGvX.
12. Ellison, Sarah. (2013). 'Diana's impossible dream', *Vanity Fair*.
13. Feiden, Douglas. 'Dodi, not Di's love, doctor stole her heart, book says', *New York Daily News*.
14. Ellison, Sarah. (2013). 'Diana's impossible dream', *Vanity Fair*.
15. Caelers, Di. 'Barnard on love, life and mercy', IOL. https://goo.gl/pF4Am1.
16. Barnard, Deirdre. (2003). *Fat, Fame and Life with Father*. Cape Town: Double Storey.
17. Caelers, Di. 'Barnard on love, life and mercy', Independent Online, 1 September 2000, www.iol.co.za. Also, Gibson, Erica. 'Heart healer, heart breaker', News24 Archives, 2 September 2001. http://www.news24.com/SouthAfrica/Heart-healer-heart-breaker-20010902.
18. Caelers, Di. 'Barnard on love, life and mercy'.
19. Gibson, Erica. 'Heart healer, heart breaker'.
20. Ibid.

21. Caelers, Di. 'Barnard on love, life and mercy'.
22. Van der Merwe, Lydia. 'Deirdre Barnard-Visser oor Parkinson se siekte: "Ek dink ek het dit"', *Sarie*, 30 June 2014.
23. Altman, Lawrence K. (2003). 'Christiaan Barnard, 78, surgeon for first heart transplant, dies', 3 September 2001. https://goo.gl/EZNaqQ.
24. 'Worldwide Christiaan Barnard Wrap 2', Associated Press Archives. www.aparchive.com.
25. Lutchinger. 'Koning van harte', *Huisgenoot*, 13 September 2001.
26. Altman, Lawrence K. (2003). 'Christiaan Barnard, 78, surgeon for first heart transplant, dies'.
27. Ibid.
28. Ibid.
29. Barnard, Marius, with Norval, Simon. (2011). *Defining Moments*. Cape Town: Zebra Press.
30. 'Worldwide Christiaan Barnard Wrap 2', Associated Press Archives.

Chapter 18

1. Alderson, Andrew. 'Barnard tried to take heart from woman while she was still alive', *The Telegraph*, 9 November 2003. https://goo.gl/2wSB46.
2. Cooper, David. (2001). 'Christiaan Barnard and his contributions to heart transplantation', *Journal of Heart and Lung Transplantation*, 20 (6), pp 599–610. https://goo.gl/c8FKPP. Also, Brink, Johan and Hassoulas, Joannis. (2009). 'The first human heart transplant and further advances in cardiac transplantation at Groote Schuur Hospital and the University of Cape Town', *Cardiovascular Journal of Africa*, 20(1), January/February. https://goo.gl/2QYwJj.
3. Altman, Lawrence. 'Christiaan Barnard, 78, surgeon for first heart transplant, dies', 3 September 2001. https://goo.gl/EZNaqQ.
4. Ibid.
5. Ibid.
6. Barnard, Christiaan, and Molloy, Bob (ed.). (1984). *The Best of Barnard*. Cape Town: Molloy Publishers.
7. Barnard, Deirdre. (2003). *Fat, Fame and Life with Father.*
8. Cooper, David (ed.). (1992). *Chris Barnard: By Those Who Know Him*. Cape Town: Vlaeberg.
9. Altman, Lawrence. 'Christiaan Barnard, 78, surgeon for first heart transplant, dies'.
10. UCT Archives.
11. Ibid.
12. Barnard, Marius with Norval, Simon. (2011) *Defining Moments*. Cape Town: Zebra Press.
13. Ibid.

14. Naudé, Johan. (2007). *Making the Cut in South Africa: A Medico Political Story.* London: The Royal Society of Medicine Press.
15. Red Cross War Memorial Children's Hospital. https://goo.gl/ZE7oWX. Also, Western Cape Government brochure on the hospital: https://goo.gl/nq3HSM.
16. Brink, Johan and Hassoulas, Joannis. (2009). 'The first human heart transplant and further advances in cardiac transplantation at Groote Schuur Hospital and the University of Cape Town', *Cardiovascular Journal of Africa*, 20 (1), January/ February. https://goo.gl/2QYwJj. Also, Chris Barnard Division of Cardiothoracic Surgery: 'Self-assessment of the decade ending December 2014'. 8 December 2014. https://goo.gl/goZwx5, and Hassoulas, Joannis. 'Transplantation of the heart: An overview of 40 years' clinical and research experience at Groote Schuur Hospital and the University of Cape Town'.
17. Fabian, J, Maher, H, et al. (2016). 'Favourable outcomes for the first 10 years of kidney and pancreas transplantation at Wits Donald Gordon Medical Centre, Johannesburg, South Africa', *South African Medical Journal*, 106(2), February, pp 172–176.
18. The Organ Donor Foundation of South Africa. https://odf.org.za/.
19. *The New York Times* Archives, 18 April 1968.
20. Ibid.
21. SA Medical Association president, Bernard Mandell, quoted in Cooper, David (ed.). (1992). *Chris Barnard: By Those Who Know Him*. Cape Town: Vlaeberg.

Epilogue

1. Zuhlke, Liesl. (2016). 'Why heart disease is on the rise in South Africa', UCT Research and Innovation, 29 September. https://goo.gl/KpfKSo.
2. World Health Organisation (WHO). *Cardiovascular Diseases (CVDs): Fact Sheet.* Updated May 2017.
3. Ibid.
4. Zuhlke, Liesl. (2016). 'Why heart disease is on the rise in South Africa'.
5. Barnard, Christiaan and Molloy, Bob (ed.). (1984). *The Best of Barnard*. Cape Town: Molloy Publishers.

Index

CPSIA information can be obtained
at www.ICGtesting.com
Printed in the USA
BVHW071731031218
534641BV00013B/909/P